This is a statistical analysis of dying from cancer in the United States during recent years based on state death rates. In effect, each model is an attempt to explain why more people die from cancer in one state compared to another.

The main focus is the role of the environment. A second focus is the role of lifestyle differences among people in the various states.

The statistical method used is called regression and is based on the idea of connections between things. Unfortunately, this method cannot prove cause and effect. It can still get us a little closer to understanding cancer.

There are models for the following cancers: lung, breast, colon, melanoma, bladder, Non-Hodgkin's lymphoma, pancreatic, adult leukemia, prostate, ovarian, uterine, cervical, stomach and liver.

By combining deaths from certain cancers together, the author discovered a predominating pattern – north. For just about all deaths from cancer, the more north we go, the more people die. The book ends when he reveals his best answer for what explains this pattern.

The author studied statistics for his doctorate in Jewish studies at Brown University. He became interested in cancer when his mother came down with the disease and eventually died of it. Originally from Brooklyn and Long Island New York, he lives four hours north in Providence Rhode Island.

In memory of my parents, Mindy and Bob, whom I loved

Table of Contents

DISCLAIMER: TOO DANGEROUS TO TRY II

INTRODUCTION: WE WANT CAUSES - WE END UP WITH CONNECTIONS 1
CHAPTER 1. CANCER AND RAIN 5
CHAPTER 2. CANCER (OF ALL TYPES EXCEPT LUNG) AND HAVING A DOG 25
CHAPTER 3. LUNG CANCER AND THE SUN 43
CHAPTER 4. BREAST CANCER AND AIR POLLUTION 55
CHAPTER 5. COLON CANCER AND NOT SEEING THE DENTIST 67
CHAPTER 6. MELANOMA AND HAVING A DOG 87
CHAPTER 7. BLADDER CANCER AND THE SUN 109
CHAPTER 8. NON-HODGKIN'S LYMPHOMA AND EARTH MAGNETISM 123
CHAPTER 9. PANCREATIC CANCER AND DRINKING WINE 135
CHAPTER 10. ADULT LEUKEMIA, MAGNETISM AND HAVING A DOG 151
CHAPTER 11. PROSTATE CANCER AND LIVING NORTH 165
CHAPTER 12. OVARIAN CANCER AND THE SUN 175
CHAPTER 13. UTERINE CANCER, AIR POLLUTION AND THE SUN 189
CHAPTER 14. CERVICAL CANCER, THE DENTIST AND AFRICAN AMERICANS 211
CHAPTER 15. STOMACH CANCER AND BEING SHORT 223
CHAPTER 16. LIVER CANCER AND FREQUENT SEX 233
CHAPTER 17. THREE SUMMARY TABLES 247
CHAPTER 18. THE EIGHT NORTHERN CANCERS 271
CHAPTER 19. WHAT EXPLAINS THE NORTH PATTERN OF CANCER? 291

SOURCES AND ACKNOWLEDGEMENTS 307

Disclaimer: Too Dangerous to Try

While we would all like to have better ideas we can use to treat cancer or to prevent it, it is not my intention here for individuals to use the ideas in this book for that purpose. It is simply too dangerous.

The work here is intended as an aspiration toward a better academic understanding of cancer based on the pattern of deaths across the United States. Despite my occasional exuberance in the text which I have not censored, neither I nor my company should be held responsible should harm come to anyone, God forbid, from attempting to apply the ideas here.

There are many reasons to be extremely cautious, some of which I will mention now. As of the time of this writing, the work here has not been peer reviewed and there could be obvious, gross errors of which I am not aware.

None of the ideas or devices that might be implied by them have been evaluated by the US government body FDA (Food and Drug Administration) for either safety or efficacy as it relates to cancer. The same holds true for equivalent authorities in other countries.

While the extreme macro focus of this research has its strengths, it far exceeds the more typical comparisons between groups such as those who have a disease and those who do not. This is a comparison between states within the United States, and it is unclear what conclusions can be solidly deduced from this kind of macro study.

The "ecological fallacy" suggests that knowledge derived from one level of analysis, that of large groups, cannot automatically be assumed to be correct for another level of analysis, that of an individual. In other words, conclusions in these studies suggesting links between environmental and lifestyle items and dying from cancer, might not be helpful for any particular individual.

As I state on numerous occasions, cause and effect cannot be definitively determined in this kind of correlational research. This is notwithstanding my best attempts to suggest at certain points that such results might have meaning for better understanding cancer.

Despite my years of work, it is in the nature of the research itself that we must conclude that the effort here is preliminary. While it serves the purpose of suggesting new ideas, it must be followed up by other kinds of research that provide more certainty that the identified connections are solid and true.

Introduction: Cancer – while we want to know causes, the best we can do is find connections.

In a given year in the United States, cancer is the second biggest death category after cardiovascular disease (heart disease and stroke together). Why do people die from cancer? What causes it? How can we prevent it? Can we do a better job in stopping people from dying who already have it?

I got interested in this topic when my mother got cancer. Well, it was actually a year after she was treated for cancer in her sinus, behind an eye. It kept coming back even though she was treated in New York at a top hospital. For the first time, I realized that it might kill her.

Was there anything I could do to help her, to save her? I know it sounds a little crazy. They spent billions on cancer already. I was not an oncologist, not a medical doctor. I was not a microbiologist or a geneticist. I did have a Ph.D. though. In Jewish studies.

I HAD learned statistics. Maybe I could use my knowledge to come up with something, something that might save her. It was worth a try. She was such a wonderful woman, a great mother. So I turned my focus. Then it was voting for the Nazis and now, I would look at dying from cancer.

I started this look at cancer back in 1997. I did not save her. My mother died two years later, may she rest in peace. By then, however, I was already interested. I have been working on this ever since. I would like to think the purpose is to perhaps help other people. What kept me going, however, was what author Alfie Kohn calls "intrinsic motivation". I got interested in the science questions.

How could I work on something so long? I figured out how while writing my dissertation at Brown University which took a few years. It taught me to work for long periods of time without positive reinforcement from others, without those outside goodies that keep people going. On this project, I largely worked on my own, which has its pros and cons. For me, it was the best thing and I can't imagine having reached this point in a different framework.

I have been working on cancer for so long that this could be my "life's work", named that by my nephew. It could turn out to be true but I am still hoping that more will come of it.

Ironically, our main interest here is in what "causes" cancer. That is the very word I am not allowed to use, however. Every science method has its pluses and minuses. The statistical method I use here cannot prove cause and effect.

It is called regression and is based on the idea of connections between things. When two things are connected, it is called a correlation. Regression can look at how three things are connected. More exactly, we are looking at one thing and we want to know if the other two are connected independently of each other.

Due to limitations in the method itself, we are unable to ever say that something causes cancer. The best we can do is to show a connection with cancer. Of course, this suggests the possibility that, if it is connected to cancer, that it might cause cancer.

In the end, we build "a case", like in the law field. If "this" is connected to cancer, then it might cause cancer. To prove it though, we have to follow up with a different kind of research that can test the possibility in a more rigorous manner.

There are many ways that this correlational research can go astray. I would say the biggest one is misspecification. I show that something is linked in a pattern with dying from cancer. While it looks like it could be a "cause", it might actually be something else that is strongly connected to what I have identified that is the true cause.

Once again here, like in law, by testing other possibilities, you build a case, that it really is this and not that. In the end, you can never be completely sure because you can't think of everything.

If this method of statistical connections between things is so limited, so flawed, then why use it? First, all science methods have their flaws including controlled experiments. Even published experimental research can lead to erroneous conclusions. This is on account of researcher bias, misinterpretations and mistakes.

The correlational method used here also has a great strength. It provides a very macro look at the pattern of dying from cancer. These models include virtually all the recorded deaths from cancer during the time period across one large country, the United States. It is a "big data" project in its essence even though its beginning predated my awareness of that concept.

It is as if we are out in space, above the atmosphere of the planet, looking down on the entire country of the United States in one view. The question is why more people are dying in states over in that part of the country as opposed to this part? What can explain this pattern? Knowing that might give us important new information about why people are dying from cancer.

What is the connection between the results in these cancer models and "reality"? I know that people die of cancer all the time and we all want to know why? That is quite real.

Unfortunately, however, we cannot directly access reality. The best we can do with these methods is to suggest a possible version of reality. This is so despite the fact that I convince myself working on each new model that it is all "the God's honest truth", reality itself.

The results change depending on how many items are in the model, which items are in. How can this be reality?

We come up with an item to test, having a dog as an example. We get numbers for that. Unfortunately, there is always error and imperfection in any attempt to represent something in number form.

Of course, ultimately, we are all limited by our own understanding of things and by our imagination. Here I came up with ideas that I was able to represent in number form. Then I was able to test them to see if they were linked with cancer. Other people would test other ideas. None of it is reality itself, partly because it is so connected to me, so much a product of my own mind.

Nevertheless, despite the obvious imperfections, the effort is worthwhile. By producing a description of one possible version of reality that these models do, they stimulate our thinking, get us closer and closer to the day when we will figure out cancer.

This study is limited to deaths from cancer in one country, the United States. While perhaps US states are also involved with gathering this data, I believe that the United States basically constitutes one statistical unit for death rates.

While much could also be learned from international comparisons between countries, there is more chance for error. This is due to the fact that they might not count things in the same way in other countries making valid comparisons more difficult. Generally speaking, I do believe that what affects cancer in one big country (like the United States) has relevance for understanding cancer in other places too.

As I mentioned, I use a simple statistical method called linear regression in these models. This technique has been around for many decades. I realize that it has fallen out of vogue but I use it here mainly because I know it best. I also happen to believe that it might be technically superior to the more popular version as it leaves the items in continuous form.

As I understand it, the main flaw of simple regression is that the results are difficult to explain. For this reason, I have invested considerable effort in presenting the results in as clear a manner as I can even for readers unfamiliar with statistics. Time will tell whether or not I have succeeded in this particular endeavor.

I have designed the chapters in such a way that the framework for each is similar to each other. While this makes for a certain repetitiveness, I have a strong hunch that there will be readers who wish to jump around to the particular cancers that interest them most.

In this way, each chapter is largely independent and able to be understood without reading the whole book in the order in which it is presented. Nevertheless, the first chapter or two are more detailed because I introduce for the first time the format I follow throughout. The chapters become more readable as they move forward as I learn from experience to express myself a little more clearly.

The bulk of the chapters are about one particular cancer, looking at the pattern of deaths by state after the actual number of deaths has been changed into a "rate". The purpose of this first change, done by the government statisticians, is so big states can be compared to small states. Big states have more deaths because there are more people.

Two chapters at the beginning and two at the end take a broader look at dying from cancer. There, various individual cancers are added together. While there are strengths and weaknesses of each view, I suspect that this aggregation adds power to the analysis due to the larger numbers.

The third chapter from the end is an interim summary of all the individual cancer models including three tables of the results. That was going to be my final chapter but, to my surprise, there was more work to do.

While I don't care to reveal the drama right now, the main result is surprising. This is not necessarily a bad thing because, Lord knows, we need some fresh thinking about this disease. More than a half million people are dying of cancer year in and year out. (In 2017, some six hundred thousand are expected to die, according to the American Cancer Society). This is just in one country, the United States.

Working so many years, I did this research and wrote up these results on cancer, ultimately, to answer the questions that I, personally, wanted to know. So at this point, when you the reader are joining me, I am humbled and grateful for your arrival. Together, may we figure out cancer a little better.

Lastly, I wish to alert the reader to a possible error in the text. When I start discussing deaths from a new cancer, I compare deaths from that cancer to all deaths from cancer as well as to deaths from all causes. Some cancers, however, only strike those of one gender such as prostate for men and for women, ovarian, uterine and cervical. Before making the above comparison, I suggest that it might be necessary to double these numbers. While this was my best guess at the time, and I decided to leave it as written, I now suspect that such a doubling might not be necessary. I am still uncertain which of the two options is correct.

Chapter 1. Cancer of All Types Together and its Link with Rain

In this chapter, I present the full cancer model identifying the four items which help to explain the pattern across the states of the United States. The question here is why is it that the death rate from cancer is higher in some states than in others?

The first explanation is older age. The higher the proportion of the population in the state that is in the "senior" category, age 65 and over, the higher the death rate from cancer.

The second explanation (in size order) is smoking. The higher the percent of the population in 1996 that said they were smokers, the higher the death rate from cancer.

The third explanation is what I call rain. It includes snow and is more properly called precipitation. The more inches of rain that come down over the course of the year in the largest city of the state, the higher the death rate from cancer.

The fourth and last explanation item is Jews. The higher the percent of the population of the state that is Jewish, the lower the death rate from cancer.

Soon, I will present the list of states for each explanation item so we can become more familiar with each before moving to the model itself which is the attempt to explain all deaths from cancer. First, however, we must start with the initial list itself of cancer death rates by state. Table 1-1 is the cancer death rate for US states (including Washington DC, counted as if it were a state and called "District" in the tables, short for District of Columbia). This is the yearly average for the three year period of 2010, 2011 and 2012.

All the cancer deaths in each state are counted and converted into a rate by dividing them by the state's population size to yield a death "rate" per hundred thousand people. In this way, the number from a large state (with more deaths, of course) can be compared in a valid manner with cancer deaths in a small state with, of course, fewer deaths.

The cancer death rate is organized in Table 1-1 from lowest to highest, Utah at about 145 deaths per hundred thousand people to West Virginia with about 321 deaths per hundred thousand.

Table 1-1 Cancer death rate by state 2010-2012
(per hundred thousand people)

State	Rate	State	Rate
Utah	144.8	Kansas	251.7
Alaska	170.6	Montana	253.0
Colorado	183.1	New Hampshire	254.0
Texas	199.2	Oregon	257.6
California	199.4	Wisconsin	259.1
District	207.5	Rhode Island	263.5
Hawaii	211.5	South Carolina	264.7
Georgia	213.6	South Dakota	265.0
New Mexico	216.3	Louisiana	267.1
Idaho	220.9	Indiana	268.7
Nevada	221.3	Michigan	270.0
Arizona	222.2	Vermont	270.7
Wyoming	222.7	Delaware	272.3
Washington	227.5	Iowa	274.4
Virginia	227.6	Missouri	275.2
Maryland	230.3	Florida	276.9
Minnesota	233.4	Tennessee	277.2
New York	233.8	Alabama	278.1
North Dakota	239.7	Oklahoma	278.3
New Jersey	245.1	Ohio	283.8
Connecticut	245.2	Mississippi	284.4
North Carolina	247.3	Pennsylvania	289.7
Illinois	247.3	Arkansas	291.8
Nebraska	248.2	Kentucky	295.3
Massachusetts	248.5	Maine	304.1
		West Virginia	320.6

People are naturally drawn to see how their state does if they live in the United States. I caution, however, that there is not so much a person might learn from this raw list before first accounting for big influences that might not be that interesting to us. As an example, older age is very much linked with dying from cancer. The original list in Table 1-1 might be heavily affected by this connection with which we are all familiar.

Now we can begin with the particular four items that help explain cancer which I present in size order, the first having the strongest effect. That would be the percent "seniors" age 65 and over in Table 1-2. The smallest percent of the state population in this age category is in Alaska (in 2006) with about 7 percent seniors. The highest is Florida with about 17% seniors. The middle area (25th on the list) is South Carolina with 13% seniors. More seniors, a higher death rate from cancer.

The second explanation item is smokers. Table 1-3 is the percent of people when polled who said they were smokers (in 1996). The smallest percent is Utah at around 16% of the population and the largest percent smokers is in Kentucky with about 32%. The middle state (number 25) is Arizona where 24% said they were smokers.

The third explanation item is rain found in Table 1-4. (It actually includes snow but, for purposes of figuring out the amount, snow in inches is first converted to liquid form). This is a yearly average of precipitation reaching the ground over a thirty year period measured in inches. It is recorded in the largest city of the state (in terms of population size) and it is this value that is used to represent the entire state, a compromise that works well in small states, less well in large states in terms of territory such as California and New York. Yearly "rain" starts at a low of about 4 inches in Nevada and goes to a high of about 62 inches a year for Louisiana. The approximate middle value for the 25th state on the list is Ohio with 37 inches a year.

The final explanation item is Jews and can be found in Table 1-5. The percent of the population that is Jewish goes from Idaho with a tenth of one percent to New York with about 9 percent. The approximate middle value for the 25th state is Washington (state) whose state population is six tenth of one percent Jewish.

The regression method assumes that explanation items are not connected with each other (correlated).

Table 1-2 Older Age.
Percent Age 65 and Over in each state (2006)

State	%	State	%
Alaska	6.8	Kentucky	12.8
Utah	8.8	New Jersey	12.9
Georgia	9.8	Kansas	12.9
Texas	9.9	Oregon	12.9
Colorado	10.0	Wisconsin	13.0
California	10.8	New York	13.1
Nevada	11.1	Oklahoma	13.2
Idaho	11.5	Nebraska	13.3
Washington	11.5	Massachusetts	13.3
Virginia	11.6	Vermont	13.3
Maryland	11.6	Missouri	13.3
Illinois	12.0	Connecticut	13.4
Minnesota	12.1	Delaware	13.4
Wyoming	12.2	Alabama	13.4
North Carolina	12.2	Ohio	13.4
Louisiana	12.2	Montana	13.8
District	12.3	Rhode Island	13.9
New Mexico	12.4	Arkansas	13.9
New Hampshire	12.4	Hawaii	14.0
Indiana	12.4	South Dakota	14.2
Mississippi	12.4	North Dakota	14.6
Michigan	12.5	Iowa	14.6
Tennessee	12.7	Maine	14.6
Arizona	12.8	Pennsylvania	15.2
South Carolina	12.8	West Virginia	15.3
		Florida	16.8

Table 1-3 Smokers. Percent Smokers (1996) in each state

State	%	State	%
Utah	15.8	Massachusetts	23.7
Hawaii	17.5	Wyoming	24.0
California	18.7	Vermont	24.2
Georgia	19.9	Delaware	24.3
Maryland	20.8	North Dakota	24.3
District	20.8	South Carolina	24.4
Minnesota	21.1	Virginia	24.6
Idaho	21.3	Oklahoma	24.6
South Dakota	21.5	Iowa	24.6
Montana	21.7	Illinois	25.1
Connecticut	22.2	Wisconsin	25.2
Alabama	22.6	Pennsylvania	25.3
Texas	22.8	North Carolina	25.7
New Mexico	22.8	New Hampshire	25.7
Kansas	22.9	Louisiana	25.8
Florida	22.9	Michigan	25.8
Nebraska	23.0	Maine	26.1
Mississippi	23.1	Alaska	26.2
Rhode Island	23.1	Arkansas	26.5
Colorado	23.5	West Virginia	27.0
Washing	23.6	Tennessee	28.0
New Jersey	23.6	Missouri	28.0
Oregon	23.6	Nevada	28.1
New York	23.6	Indiana	28.8
Arizona	23.7	Ohio	29.5
		Kentucky	31.7

Table 1-4 rain.

Inches of rain over the whole year in the largest city of the state (including snow converted to liquid).

State	Inches	State	Inches
Nevada	4.1	Missouri	37.6
Arizona	7.7	District	38.6
New Mexico	8.9	Indiana	39.9
Montana	11.6	Maryland	40.8
Idaho	12.1	Delaware	40.8
Wyoming	14.4	Pennsylvania	41.4
California	14.8	North Carolina	41.4
Alaska	15.9	Massachusetts	41.5
Colorado	16.1	West Virginia	42.5
Utah	16.2	Virginia	43.2
North Dakota	19.5	New Jersey	44.0
Hawaii	22.0	Connecticut	44.1
South Dakota	23.9	Maine	44.3
Minnesota	28.3	Kentucky	44.6
Kansas	29.3	Rhode Island	45.5
Nebraska	29.9	Texas	46.1
Michigan	32.6	New York	47.3
Wisconsin	32.9	Georgia	50.8
Iowa	33.1	Arkansas	50.9
Oklahoma	33.4	South Carolina	51.5
Vermont	34.5	Tennessee	52.1
Illinois	35.8	Alabama	54.6
Oregon	36.3	Mississippi	55.4
New Hampshire	36.4	Florida	55.9
Ohio	36.6	Louisiana	61.9
Washington	37.2		

Table 1-5 Jews.
Percent of the state population that is Jewish (1996)

Montana	.1	Maine	.6
Idaho	.1	Texas	.6
Wyoming	.1	New Hampshire	.8
North Dakota	.1	Minnesota	.9
South Dakota	.1	Vermont	1.0
West Virginia	.1	Michigan	1.1
Arkansas	.1	Virginia	1.1
Mississippi	.1	Ohio	1.2
Utah	.2	Missouri	1.2
Iowa	.2	Georgia	1.2
Oklahoma	.2	Nevada	1.4
South Carolina	.2	Colorado	1.4
Alabama	.2	Rhode Island	1.6
Indiana	.3	Arizona	1.8
North Carolina	.3	Delaware	1.9
Kentucky	.3	Illinois	2.3
Tennessee	.3	Pennsylvania	2.7
Nebraska	.4	California	2.9
Louisiana	.4	Connecticut	3.0
New Mexico	.5	Maryland	4.2
Alaska	.5	Massachusetts	4.4
Hawaii	.6	Florida	4.5
Kansas	.6	District	4.6
Wisconsin	.6	New Jersey	5.5
Oregon	.6	New York	9.1
Washington	.6		

If such connections are too high, the model results might be unreliable leading to sometimes erroneous conclusions. In reality, items ARE commonly connected to each other to some degree.

The first test for such (bad) connectedness is statistical significance (a problem at the "two star" level of .01). The second test is the actual size of the connection from .1 to .99. The larger the connection, the greater the chance of a potential problem. The rule I learned for a problem size of a correlation is anything above .6. In recent years, however, I have become more strict seeking a much lower number for greater certainty that the model results are valid.

In Table 1-6, I present correlations for the cancer model. (In subsequent tables, I put the correlations at the end of the model page. Here the model is divided into two tables, the main model being in the next table, Table 1-7). The focus is on the four explanation items themselves. I also include the item in focus, in this case, death rates from cancer, in order to show the simple link between each item with cancer death rates for purposes of general interest.

This checking for "too high" interconnectedness plays a large role for deciding whether or not items linked to cancer should be included in the final model. While cancer is linked to a multitude of items, it may not be included in this final model if it is also linked, often rather randomly, to some other item in the model.

Looking at correlations in Table 1-6, cancer is linked in a simple way with three out of the four items. The highest is between older age (age 65 plus) and cancer with a positive correlation of about .77. More importantly, the four items are largely uncorrelated with each other based on the low numbers and lack of signficance with the exception of rain and age65 which has a correlation of about .3 one star (the .05 level), generally still low and at least not two stars (the .01 level) for significance. To myself, I refer to these correlations as "pretty clean" meaning close to uncorrelated, fulfilling the requirements of the regression method and paving the way to move on now to the final regression model after being convinced that the results there have at least passed this early test.

I present the final cancer model in Table 1-7. In the box on top, we find the Adjusted R Square. This is a number representation of the total portion of the pattern of cancer death rates across the 51 "states" that the model succeeds in explaining. This is .884 or 88.4 percent of the pattern. This is .884 or 88.4 percent of the pattern.

Table 1-6 cancer correlations: (all kinds of cancer)

		AGE65IN6	SMOKRS96	RAIN2	PJEWS96	CAN1012
AGE65IN6	Pearson Correlation	1	.200	.305*	.104	.769**
	Sig. (2-tailed)	.	.160	.029	.466	.000
	N	51	51	51	51	51
SMOKRS96	Pearson Correlation	.200	1	.254	-.163	.594**
	Sig. (2-tailed)	.160	.	.073	.252	.000
	N	51	51	51	51	51
RAIN2	Pearson Correlation	.305*	.254	1	.199	.557**
	Sig. (2-tailed)	.029	.073	.	.160	.000
	N	51	51	51	51	51
PJEWS96	Pearson Correlation	.104	-.163	.199	1	-.129
	Sig. (2-tailed)	.466	.252	.160	.	.367
	N	51	51	51	51	51
CAN1012	Pearson Correlation	.769**	.594**	.557**	-.129	1
	Sig. (2-tailed)	.000	.000	.000	.367	.
	N	51	51	51	51	51

*. Correlation is significant at the 0.05 level (2-tailed).
**. Correlation is significant at the 0.01 level (2-tailed).

Table 1-7 The Model for All Deaths from Cancer (2010-2012): The Role of Rain (more deaths).

Model Summary

Model	R	R Square	Adjusted R Square	Std. Error of the Estimate
1	.945[a]	.893	.884	11.8518

a. Predictors: (Constant), PJEWS96, AGE65IN6, SMOKRS96, RAIN2

Coefficients[a]

Model		Unstandardized Coefficients		Standardized Coefficients	t	Sig.
		B	Std. Error	Beta		
1	(Constant)	-40.224	17.601		-2.285	.027
	AGE65IN6	12.943	1.065	.622	12.150	.000
	SMOKRS96	4.289	.620	.357	6.914	.000
	RAIN2	.774	.130	.317	5.968	.000
	PJEWS96	-3.924	1.000	-.199	-3.925	.000

a. Dependent Variable: CAN1012

Now we move to the main box which includes the actual resulting model in number form. First is the important matter of statistical significance. In a general way, I use it as a way of assessing the solidness of the connections that were discovered in the model.

In a more technical sense, it is really a way of deciding how confident we can be that the connection discovered here between these two sets of numbers might be present in the broader population that interests us. In other words, we are examining here a particular set of deaths from cancer which occurred during a three year period and their link with items such as inches of rain which fell during a particular 30 year period.

While it is nice to find a connection between these two sets of things, we are actually interested to know a broader question. Would it also be the case that rain is related to dying from cancer if we used cancer deaths from another set of years? Would it be the case if we used inches of rain from another set of years? Would this connection remain true if we looked at deaths from cancer in Europe? While there is no way to be sure, if the statistical significance test result is strong suggesting a "solid" connection between the items, the chances are higher that this connection might show up in a different context as well.

In this particular research, there is an opposing argument that could also be made. We have no need to consider the matter of statistical significance because we are actually dealing here with not a mere sample of deaths from cancer during the three year period but, ultimately all the deaths! Assuming there are no or few mistakes in the record keeping, the numbers in Table 1-1 are actually not a sample but the entire population – all of the deaths from cancer (after being converted into a death "rate" per hundred thousand people). Seen this way, we can dispense with statistical significance which is an attempt to assess the reliability of this so called sample and how it relates to the larger population. This IS the population – all the deaths.

Between these two choices, while there are merits for both, I have decided to focus on statistical significance as one more way of ensuring that the connections I include in the model are "solid" ones. Of course, I am highly influenced in this decision by convention as well. To further ensure such "solidness", all connection in these cancer models use the more stringent cutoff of better than .01 meaning the chance of our sample not being part of the population is less than one percent.

In the main model box, there are three columns related to the statistical significance test. The Standard Error column I have always ignored viewing it as redundant. The t column is also used for statistical significance and needs to be over 2 in size. The Sig. column is the general one I most use. Aiming for better than "the .01 level", the best score in this column is .000.

Now we are ready to look at the model box in Table 1-7 for deaths from cancer in general. First we check the statistical significance. In the last column "Sig.", all four values are lower than .01. The second column from the right called "t" gives a bit more detail on how successful the significance test actually is. Any value of t that is 2 or over is satisfactory. All four of these numbers are well over 2, the largest being older age with a value of more than 12. For Smokers, the t value is almost 7 so we can be quite confident that there is a connection between the percent of smokers in a state and deaths from cancer.

Perhaps it pays to repeat our uncertainty on two matters even after having established a "solid" link between smoking and dying from cancer. First, we can never be entirely sure that it is the smoking of smokers that causes more cancer deaths in a state. Second, we are even unable to be certain that it is the smokers themselves who are more likely to die even though we know that smoking is related to dying from cancer. In this case, such is probably the truth, however. It shows up in the model that smoking is related to cancer and this probably is because people who smoke are the ones "significantly" more likely to die from this disease.

Now we are ready to move to the size of the effects on cancer death rates of each of these connected items shown in Table 1-7. I always list the items in size order which can be seen in the third column from the right in the lower box titled "Beta". I will now show how these Beta numbers can be used to show the relative size of each effect because these numbers can be directly compared to each other.

First is the portion of the "variance explained" by each item. In this first way, we assume that these results explain the entire pattern, untrue of course, because it explains only 88.4% of the pattern. Adding the four values in the Beta column (ignoring the negative sign and the decimal point) makes 622+357+317+199=1495. 622/1495 equals about 41.6%. This is the part of the explained portion that the model succeeds in identifying that can be attributed to age. 357/1495 is about 23.9%, the portion of the model's explanation that is attributed to smokers. Rain is 317/1495 = 21.2 percent, the portion the model explains that can be attributed to rain. Lastly is Jews: 199/1495 = 13.3 percent, the part of the explained portion of cancer death rates that can be attributed to Jews (a lower cancer death rate due to the negative sign).

Next, we can use the same numbers to determine the portion of the **total** explanation of cancer death rates that can be attributed to these four items. If the Beta of the four items adds to 1495 (without decimals and negative signs) and this represents 88.4% of the total explanation, then 100% of the explanation would total to: 1495/88.4=x/100. 149500=88.4x. x=149500/88.4=1691.18. Dividing each Beta value by that number should yield the actual portion of the total explanation of cancer deaths attributable to each item.

For age, it is 622/1691.18 = 36.8 percent. For smokers, it is 357/1691.18 = 21.1 percent. For rain, it is 317/1691.18 = 18.7 percent and for percent Jews, it is 199/1691.18 = 11.8 percent. The model for cancer deaths suggests, then, that "smoking" accounts for 21.1% or a little over a fifth of the total pattern, the explanation, for what explains how cancer deaths vary by state across the United States during the years 2010-2012.

Now we can move in the lower box of Table 1-7 to the fifth column from the right, B, which is the model equation itself. By writing it out and putting in the value for each state, we should get the value for that state of cancer deaths. Of course, this equation comes from the actual numbers (of cancer death rates) for all the states and represents it in a general form which might prove useful to us in the future.

As an example, I will do this for one state, New York, the state of my birth. Here, we have to be aware of the signs (plus or minus). Minus 40.224 + [12.943 times percent age 65, value for New York in Table 1-2] + [4.289 times percent smokers, value for New York in Table 1-3] + [.774 times yearly inches of rain, value for New York in Table 1-4], minus [3.924 times percent Jews, value for New York in Table 1-5]. This is -40.224 + [(12.943)(13.1)] + [(4.289)(23.6)] + [(.774)(47.25)] - [(3.924)(9.1)]. -40.224 + 169.55 + 101.22 + 36.57 - 35.71 = 231.41.

Now we can compare this to the actual cancer death rate for New York in Table 1-1 which is 233.8. The equation suggested a value of 231.4 whereas the actual death rate is 233.8. This is quite close showing how successful the model is based on all 51 values in coming up with a shorthand way for summarizing the cancer death rate in the United States across all the states.

This equation for representing the cancer death rate might be useful in two ways. If we have the values for the four items with which cancer death rates are linked, we can use the equation to predict cancer death rates in different places, even foreign countries assuming that the pattern in the US would apply (more or less). The equation represents a general "key". I make use of it in this project for "customizing" the death rate model in order to help determine (in a more meaningful way than the general death rates in Table 1-1) which places have low cancer death rates. This should become clearer when I actually do these calculations based on this model of all cancer death rates.

The final column in the lower box of Table 1-7 is Std. Error, Standard Error. I do not make reference to it because it is used to calculate statistical significance and, is, therefore, redundant.

In this section, I will try to summarize what we learn from this statistical model of cancer deaths in the United States. Some of the comments are my own opinions and are thus, not as purely "scientific". While keeping that in mind, the discussion is important to add plausibility to the findings even though there is more room for disagreement at this stage.

As I stated before, there is no way to be certain about "who" is doing the dying from the model result. All that we know is that more people are dying from cancer (per population size) the more senior citizens there are in a state. We cannot be sure that it is the seniors themselves who are dying. Here, I make the assumption that it IS seniors. If it is true that the higher the percent of senior there are, the more deaths from cancer there are, this is because seniors, those in the age category of 65 years old or more, are dying in greater numbers when compared to the entire population.

The same applies to smokers, an example I gave earlier. While we can't know from sure if it is the smokers themselves who are more likely to die from cancer, I again assume that if "smokers" is linked with deaths from cancer, it is because smokers are the ones who are significantly more likely to die from cancer.

The same would be true for the rather enigmatic result about Jews and fewer deaths from cancer. If there are fewer cancer deaths in states with more Jews, then I presume this is because, compared with the population as a whole, Jews are less likely to die from cancer.

Of course, other explanations are possible which would have to be carefully checked to see if they are plausible. As Jews might typically live in larger cities, perhaps fewer people in large cities die from cancer because those areas might have better hospitals. Here, typically, I just assume the simple explanation that it is Jews themselves who are less likely to die of cancer rather than the more complicated possibility. The "why" is left as an open question about which we might speculate.

What is the meaning of these findings and what might they teach us about cancer in general? Of course, to die from cancer, you first have to get it. I focus on deaths because it is more definitive than disease "incidence" and I assume there is less "error" for cancer deaths compared with cancer incidence.

First is the link between older age and cancer. It is interesting that many of these models highlight the age 65 age category as most strongly connected with dying from cancer rather than the age 85 category, another I have tested. It is at this age, 65, when the dying from cancer, apparently picks up in velocity.

First is the obvious point we all know that dying in general is concentrated among older people. Of course, some young people also die but we are far less surprised to hear than an older person has died due to this concentration of dying in this age category. Cancer is a large category in the list of death rates, at least 20 percent of all deaths. It seems not surprising at all that older people would also be more likely to die from cancer. Here again, there are exceptions with specific kinds of cancer such as stomach cancer and pancreatic cancer in women. Children get leukemia as well (but childhood leukemia is not examined in this work). Generally speaking, however, cancer is, indeed, a "disease of aging", as it is firmly understood to be. I once heard a lecture on that subject at Harvard but the details escape me now.

Why is dying from cancer linked with older age? I am not an expert who might be able to provide a good answer. One idea might be more senescent cells (that have stopped making copies of themselves) which are more prone to becoming cancerous. My own idea has to do with the slower speed of the cell cycle as we age which leaves open the result of the new copy to more errors (mutations) which end up as cancer.

If the link between dying from cancer and older age is so well known, why have it in the model? While it at least does confirm what we already know, perhaps of some value, the main reason to have age in the model is as a "control". While we, of course, want to learn things that are new, if we do not first account for the link with age, we would never be able to get a clear look at what else might be linked with cancer. After accounting for the well known link with age, what else might explain the pattern of cancer deaths across the United States?

It is a similar story with the second item, a link between cancer and smoking. Of several variations I tried, "percent smokers" works best and makes it to the final model. More percent smokers in the state, more deaths from cancer. Again here, we can assume this is so because it is smokers themselves who are doing the "extra" dying from cancer. We further assume that this is not because they were less likely to go to college, as an alternative possibility, but, rather, because smoking itself is so physically harmful that it causes them to get cancer and to die from it. (I reach a somewhat different conclusion later on in the book, however). While, from the perspective of today, this all seems self-evident, we must remember back to before the 1960s when they first determined the link between smoking and lung cancer.

With so many new findings in this research, it is somewhat reassuring that something we all "know" that is linked with cancer ends up being an item in the final model. A twist awaits us about smoking in future models, however.

Skipping now to item number four is the last minute finding that percent Jews is linked with fewer deaths from cancer. This is quite a surprise because, being Jewish myself, many of the people I know who have died from cancer happen to have been Jewish, including my own mother, may she rest in peace. This result is telling us, however, that, of all the many connections I tried, this one, between the size of the Jewish population of a state and cancer deaths, is so distinctive that it can be discerned with a statistical test. To repeat, I interpret this result to mean not that Jews do not die from cancer but rather that Jews are "significantly" less likely to die from cancer compared to the general population.

What might account for this result is quite a mystery. In this work, I tend to discount physical or genetic differences between groups in the US population partly because I do not have the background to do biological or genetic research. My general sense is, however, that any such differences are so slight that a more productive place to look for an explanation is variations between groups in terms of lifestyle. Actually, in a late breaking development, I might have fallen upon a portion of the explanation for why the percent of the state population that is Jewish happens to be linked with fewer cancer deaths in that state. I will save it for an upcoming model in the following chapter whose results help to solve this mystery, at least in part.

Lastly is the premiere result of the model on cancer, something probably genuinely new: rain. The more precipitation there is over the course of the year in the largest city of the state (a thirty year average), the more deaths from cancer there are in that state. Cancer is linked with rain!

As for why, I am on my own here and I will offer a few ideas. First, rain is moisture and bacteria love moisture, need moisture, to grow and reproduce. Cancer might thrive in the wetter conditions where there is more rain because increased bacterial growth might be a key component in the switching of normal cells to cancer ones. Bacterial overgrowth in the gut can interfere with the immune response there, as one example unrelated to cancer.

Too many bacteria, encouraged by the more moist conditions of additional rain, might somehow interfere with the cell copying process leaving too many cells damaged, without having successfully made it through replication. Furthermore, perhaps this posited overgrowth of bacteria might interfere with the cell killing mechanism of apoptosis. This would leave too many damaged cells around in the system taking up too much space and crowding out healthy cells which would not have enough room to do their work.

Thinking about qualities of rain unrelated to moisture, there are other possibilities as well. I will mention two such additional ideas. Increased gamma radiation is linked with thunderstorms. It is a relatively new piece of information that terrestrial thunderstorms with their lightning give off gamma radiation. Furthermore, I read that rain brings down with it additional radiation to the ground from higher elevations in the atmosphere. Perhaps this additional gamma radiation that accompanies rain from both sources might help to cause cancer.

Lastly is the electrical component of rain (and thunderstorms), the effect of such weather disturbances on the electrical signature of the air as well as inside the body. This topic of air electricity is very confusing with the common insistence on separating charged air particles of a negative and positive charge. From my own experimentation using a "body voltage meter", I have first concluded that the body takes on the electrical signature of the air. Body electricity goes down during rain by about half. Perhaps this reduced level of total body electricity during rain might promote cancer.

One additional clarification is necessary. I have tested many variations of "rain" (which of course, here, includes snow in liquid form for measuring as well as even the tad bit of dew). Such items related to rain include measures for snow, thunderstorm days, lightning, dew point, and humidity. Despite all the tests, it is "rain" in inches over the course of the year that is the one that works best in the model for explaining cancer. This additional information might help in the sorting between various possibilities regarding the why - why rain is linked with cancer.

Lastly, we dare not leave the model in its current form, based as it is on actual cancer death rates in a given year across all the states. There is a way of "customizing" the model for different purposes with the goal of making it more meaningful, more illuminating. The government statisticians provide one example of this: age-adjusted numbers of cancer death rates. Why do they do this? As it is well known that dying from cancer is so strongly linked with being "older", it allows us to see the pattern AFTER accounting for that fact.

This model of cancer deaths well confirms that age is related to dying from cancer with the finding that age 65 explains 36.8% of the entire pattern across the states, over a third. It is nice to have a look at the pattern after accounting for that rather well known connection. The government age adjustment is probably better than my own but the point is still largely the same. What motivates this work, however, is the desire to have a closer look. How about the other 63.2 percent of the pattern, a clear majority? What might explain this part, the rest of the pattern? This is where the current model provides a new look.

We can achieve a clearer view of cancer deaths across the United States by largely eliminating the effects of all three of the "people" descriptions. As the government does with age, it provides a look at the list of cancer deaths by state after an age adjustment. Here now, we want to achieve the same thing by adjusting not only for age but for two other items, smokers and Jews.

There is a way of doing this while still using the original equation for cancer deaths in Table 1-7. We can "zero out" the "people" effects above by replacing each state's value with an average for all the states, the mean. When the computer program works through the equation to come up with a value for each state, by having the value as the same, it eliminates entirely the difference between states, in effect largely nullifying that item. We do this for all three items we wish to set aside leaving only the one item we wish to vary.

We can do this now, this manipulation, to gain a clearer view for the cancer deaths equation from Table 1-7, the B column. We will put in mean values for age 65, smokers, and Jews leaving only the environmental factor of "rain" to vary and affect our prediction of cancer death rates by state.

In the statistical software package SPSS 11 for Mac OS X, we can find the mean values for the three items whose impact we desire to "zero out" from the pull down menu - analyze, descriptive statistics, descriptives. The means, which happen to be percents, are as follows: age65 12.653, smokers 23.986, and Jews 1.349. With the one remaining item we DO wish to vary, rain, we let it vary by adding the name of the item which tells the program to calculate the equation plugging in the rain value for each individual state.

We do this from the data file finding transform, and then compute and filling in the boxes. I will call the new item canrain. Canrain = -40.224 + (12.943 * 12.653) + (4.289 * 23.986) + (.774 * rain2) - (2.924 * 1.349). This is in the order of the way the equation is listed in the B column of Table 1-7 with the first number being the constant, the second, the age number multiplied by the mean value for age, the smokers number multiplied by the mean value for smokers, the rain number multiplied by the actual value for rain for each state, putting in the name of the item, and the Jews value multiplied by the mean value for Jews (being careful to accurately represent the minus sign (because the more Jews, the FEWER the cancer deaths). Now we run canrain. May we have luck.

Canrain can now be found in Table 1-8. This, in my estimation, is the most meaningful view of state level cancer deaths in the United States based on actual state death rates in 2010-2012 but reconfigured to show the predicted death rate by state with the only relevant part of the finding changing by state: rain. Of course, the specific order of this list of what I call "predicted" death rates is a variation of the actual ones after accounting for differences between states that are not of first order interest (including older age, smokers and Jews).

In calculating this new view of cancer deaths, we allow to vary the one environmental item in the model, rain. Of course, the ordering of this list is, thus, identical to the rain list in Table 1-4.

So far, we can reach the simple conclusion then, that the most relevant environmental factor affecting deaths from cancer as revealed in the equation of cancer deaths in a recent year is how much rain a place gets over the course of the year. The more rain, the more cancer deaths.

Apparently, the less rain there is, the fewer the cancer deaths as well. After accounting for the effects of age, smokers, and Jews, Nevada, being the state with the least rain (based on Las Vegas) should have the fewest cancer deaths per population size. (As I mentioned, looking at the actual rain numbers in Table 1-4 is another view of the same thing). Table 1-8 Canrain, however, gives the predicted death rate from cancer in the state (again, after accounting for the other items in the model, largely neutralizing their effect).

Comparing the cancer death rate in the highest state (269.0 per hundred thousand, the death rate in Nevada (224.3) is only about 83 percent as large. 269.0/100=224/x. 22400+269.0x. x=22400/269.0. x=83.27. If death rates in the lowest cancer state Nevada are only some 83 percent as high compared to the highest death rate state, this means that death rates in the lowest cancer state of Nevada are [(100-83.27137)= 16.729 or] about 16.7% lower in the lowest cancer state compared to the highest. This is based only on how much rain they get there (very little, a desert after all). So far, we have a simple conclusion from the model of all cancer death rates in the United States after accounting for the differences between people in each state. Rain is bad for cancer.

Table 1-8 [canrain] cancer rain. Best view predicted death rate from cancer of all kinds in 2010-2012. Here, we set aside the three effects of older age (more deaths), smokers (more deaths) and Jews (fewer deaths) to see the impact more clearly of rain (more deaths).

Nevada	224.3	Missouri	250.2
Arizona	227.1	District	251.0
New Mexico	228.0	Indiana	252.0
Montana	230.1	Maryland	252.7
Idaho	230.5	Delaware	252.7
Wyoming	232.3	Pennsylvania	253.2
California	232.6	North Carolina	253.2
Alaska	233.4	Massachusetts	253.3
Colorado	233.6	West Virginia	254.0
Utah	233.6	Virginia	254.5
North Dakota	236.2	New Jersey	255.2
Hawaii	238.2	Connecticut	255.3
South Dakota	239.6	Maine	255.4
Minnesota	243.0	Kentucky	255.6
Kansas	243.8	Rhode Island	256.4
Nebraska	244.2	Texas	256.8
Michigan	246.4	New York	257.7
Wisconsin	246.6	Georgia	260.4
Iowa	246.8	Arkansas	260.5
Oklahoma	246.9	South Carolina	261.0
Vermont	247.8	Tennessee	261.5
Illinois	248.9	Alabama	263.4
Oregon	249.2	Mississippi	264.0
New Hampshire	249.3	Florida	264.4
Ohio	249.5	Louisiana	269.0
Washington	249.9		

Chapter 2. All Deaths from Cancer with the Exception of Lung Cancer: A Link with having a Dog

In the total cancer model above, not all cancers of various kinds are the same in size. Some have more deaths, some fewer deaths. It is perhaps well known that lung cancer is the primary cancer in terms of size. While the yearly death rate from cancer in general during the time 2010-2012 is about 248.1 deaths per hundred thousand, the yearly death rate of this biggest kind of cancer, lung cancer, is 68.7. 68.749/248.122 = .277. Of all deaths from cancer, lung cancer represents 27.7 percent of the total, over a quarter from just this one kind. This leaves a remainder of 72.3 percent as the portion of cancer deaths from kinds of cancer other than lung cancer.

On a hunch, not really able to verbalize why I suspect that lung cancer might be unusually distinctive, I decided now to remove lung cancer deaths from the above total deaths from cancer leaving all deaths from cancer minus lung cancer. The focus is still on the general question of "cancer" but now without cancer of the lungs.

This is the next model to see if there are new things we can learn by looking at cancer in this way. Yes, after that, I have little choice but to do a separate model for lung cancer to look at this "elephant in the room" as well, but later. I will call this model "cancer without lung".

Following the presentation in the full cancer model, I will first introduce the items in the model briefly. Then the actual lists of each item will be shown so the reader will have a chance to become acquainted with the items up close (that are related to cancer without lung). Next, I will discuss the correlations between the items to show that there is little connection between them, a requirement for a valid model. After that, I will present the actual model for cancer without lung.

Finally, like for the whole cancer model, I will decide which manipulations of the model make sense for giving us the most meaningful view of the pattern of deaths from cancer without lung. Of course, I will highlight the differences with the full cancer model to emphasize what is new in this work done with the change of removing lung cancer and looking at the remaining portion of the 72% of cancer deaths that do not involve cancer of the lungs.

For this model, cancer without lung, there are four items that explain the pattern. The first in size (biggest) is age 65. More people in the state who are age 65 or older, more deaths from cancer without lung.

Table 2-0 canolung (cancer no lung).

Cancer death rates in 2010-2012 after removing the biggest cancer, lung cancer deaths (per hundred thousand people).

Utah	121.5	New Jersey	184.5
Alaska	122.8	Montana	186.0
Colorado	141.6	South Carolina	187.0
Texas	147.6	Indiana	187.6
Georgia	152.0	Tennessee	188.2
California	154.5	Louisiana	188.2
Nevada	158.5	Oregon	188.4
District	161.7	Rhode Island	189.6
Hawaii	162.2	Delaware	189.7
Virginia	163.6	Missouri	190.1
Arizona	165.9	Wisconsin	190.4
Washington	167.1	Kentucky	191.1
Idaho	167.5	Alabama	192.2
New Mexico	168.7	Michigan	192.4
Maryland	169.4	Oklahoma	193.1
Wyoming	169.7	South Dakota	193.8
North Carolina	172.6	Vermont	195.6
New York	173.7	Arkansas	196.3
Minnesota	175.8	Mississippi	197.6
North Dakota	178.7	Florida	197.6
Illinois	179.1	Ohio	199.8
Massachusetts	181.4	Iowa	199.9
Kansas	181.5	Pennsylvania	212.1
New Hampshire	182.0	Maine	214.8
Connecticut	182.3	West Virginia	217.6
Nebraska	183.0		

Second is a new item: geomagnetism, the size of the Earth's magnetic field on the ground at the location of the largest city in the state.

This is based not on an actual measurement but rather a model which predicts the size of the magnetic field at different locations across the Earth. I constructed these numbers using an online calculator created by the government agency which specializes in Earth magnetism, USGS, The US Geological Survey.

In a rough description of how magnetism changes in our Northern hemisphere, Earth magnetism increases as we move from locations near the equator to locations further north near the pole. This happens to be the geomagnetic pole rather than the geographic pole, the place where Santa lives. The higher the level of geomagnetism at the location of the largest city of the state, the more deaths from cancer without lung in that state (per population size).

The third item is rain. The more rain (precipitation, which includes snow) over the course of the year in the largest city of the state, the more deaths from cancer without lung.

Item four is another new one, a connection with having a dog. The more households with one or more dogs living there (as a percent of all the households in the state), the more deaths from cancer without lung.

I should note right now that this saddens me greatly because, while I never had a pet growing up, I know full well how people love their pets and I much prefer to find that things people love are actually healthy leading to less disease and longer life. I even feel the need to apologize for such a troubling finding. I hope it is clear that, while I did come up with the idea to check pets for their health effects, how the model came out was largely beyond my control.

Moving now to the state lists for each items, we begin with Table 2-1 Percent Age 65, a repeat from the previous model. The senior population as a percent goes from a low in Alaska of 6.8 percent to a high in Florida of 16.8 percent. The mean (average value) is 12.653 percent - all the states added together and divided by the number of states (51 being 50 states plus the capital city of Washington DC called on the list "District", short for District of Colombia). For clarity, Washington called Washing (due to an eight character maximum), is Washington state on the west coast of the US.

Table 2-1 Older Age.
Percent Age 65 and Over in each state (2006)

State	%	State	%
Alaska	6.8	Kentucky	12.8
Utah	8.8	New Jersey	12.9
Georgia	9.8	Kansas	12.9
Texas	9.9	Oregon	12.9
Colorado	10.0	Wisconsin	13.0
California	10.8	New York	13.1
Nevada	11.1	Oklahoma	13.2
Idaho	11.5	Nebraska	13.3
Washington	11.5	Massachusetts	13.3
Virginia	11.6	Vermont	13.3
Maryland	11.6	Missouri	13.3
Illinois	12.0	Connecticut	13.4
Minnesota	12.1	Delaware	13.4
Wyoming	12.2	Alabama	13.4
North Carolina	12.2	Ohio	13.4
Louisiana	12.2	Montana	13.8
District	12.3	Rhode Island	13.9
New Mexico	12.4	Arkansas	13.9
New Hampshire	12.4	Hawaii	14.0
Indiana	12.4	South Dakota	14.2
Mississippi	12.4	North Dakota	14.6
Michigan	12.5	Iowa	14.6
Tennessee	12.7	Maine	14.6
Arizona	12.8	Pennsylvania	15.2
South Carolina	12.8	West Virginia	15.3
		Florida	16.8

Table 2-2 is Geomagnetism which is one of many items I call "north south" varying quite closely with latitude. Geomagnetism in the large country of the United States varies from a lower level (number) in the south of the country to a higher number in the north. The lowest value is in Hawaii, by far the most southern US state, much more south on the map compared to Florida. It is somewhat surprising that the highest value for geomagnetism is not in Alaska, the most northern state by far but rather in Minnesota. This is probably due to the fact that the location of Minnesota is closer to the geomagnetic pole which is in a different location than the geographic north pole. Geomagnetism of the entire state is represented by the calculated value for the location of the largest city of the state.

The third item is what I call "rain" in inches per year. It actually also includes snow in liquid form before adding it to the total. The more formal name is precipitation. Again here, it is the value for the largest city of the state which roughly represents rain in the entire state. The least rain is in Nevada with around 4 inches per year in Las Vegas. The most is in Louisiana with around 62 inches per year in New Orleans.

The second place for most rain is Miami Florida, with around 56 inches. West Palm Beach in Palm Beach County has even more but in keeping with the rules for all the states, it must be Miami that we use, the largest city, metro area. West Palm Beach might actually have more rain than New Orleans but, again, in keeping with the rules for all the states, it is Louisiana that is designated the rainiest rather than Florida. Conversely, Key West Florida has much less rain than other parts of Florida but Florida here is represented by the city of Miami. The mean value for rain across all the states in the country is 34.9039 inches or about 35 inches a year.

The fourth and last item is dog, households with one or more dogs living there. It varies from a low of about 7 percent of households in "District", (Washington DC, District of Columbia). (Perhaps I should note that New York is the second lowest for percent of households with a dog at about 22 percent). The state with the highest percent of households with a dog is Wyoming with about 48 percent of households having a dog. The mean value for having a dog is 32.406 percent. This suggests that there is a dog in about one in three American households based on these state numbers.

Table 2-2 [geomag08]

Earth magnetism on the ground in the largest city of the state (calculated using a USGS online calculator in 2008). Measured in nanoTeslas.

State	nT	State	nT
Hawaii	35194.6	Rhode Island	52811.3
Florida	45078.7	Connecticut	52836.4
California	47745.3	Kentucky	52860.3
Louisiana	48325.3	Massachusetts	53011.3
Arizona	48534.1	Colorado	53014.7
Nevada	49545.2	Oregon	53456.0
Alabama	49669.4	New Hampshire	53462.5
Mississippi	49770.6	Kansas	53494.6
Texas	49899.2	Missouri	53505.5
South Carolina	50193.6	Idaho	53595.8
New Mexico	50259.9	Maine	53618.4
Georgia	50378.6	Indiana	53769.0
North Carolina	50851.0	Wyoming	53860.4
North Dakota	50851.0	Vermont	54102.7
Arkansas	51219.9	Ohio	54153.8
Tennessee	51411.4	Nebraska	54352.1
Oklahoma	51449.4	Washington	54573.1
Delaware	52217.7	Michigan	54746.7
Virginia	52256.3	Illinois	54816.2
District	52322.1	Iowa	54818.9
Maryland	52487.7	Wisconsin	55388.5
Pennsylvania	52568.4	Montana	55629.6
West Virginia	52647.5	South Dakota	55828.4
Utah	52714.4	Alaska	55876.7
New York	52728.4	Minnesota	56293.8
New Jersey	52789.0		

Table 2-3 rain.

Average inches of rain falling in the largest city of the state over the course of the year. (Includes snow converted to liquid).

State	Inches	State	Inches
Nevada	4.1	Missouri	37.6
Arizona	7.7	District	38.6
New Mexico	8.9	Indiana	39.9
Montana	11.6	Maryland	40.8
Idaho	12.1	Delaware	40.8
Wyoming	14.4	Pennsylvania	41.4
California	14.8	North Carolina	41.4
Alaska	15.9	Massachusetts	41.5
Colorado	16.1	West Virginia	42.5
Utah	16.2	Virginia	43.2
North Dakota	19.5	New Jersey	44.0
Hawaii	22.0	Connecticut	44.1
South Dakota	23.9	Maine	44.3
Minnesota	28.3	Kentucky	44.6
Kansas	29.3	Rhode Island	45.5
Nebraska	29.9	Texas	46.1
Michigan	32.6	New York	47.3
Wisconsin	32.9	Georgia	50.8
Iowa	33.1	Arkansas	50.9
Oklahoma	33.4	South Carolina	51.5
Vermont	34.5	Tennessee	52.1
Illinois	35.8	Alabama	54.6
Oregon	36.3	Mississippi	55.4
New Hampshire	36.4	Florida	55.9
Ohio	36.6	Louisiana	61.9
Washington	37.2		

2-4 dog.
Percent of households in a state with a dog. (One or more).

State	%	State	%
District	6.9	Alaska	34.0
New York	21.9	Washington	34.0
Massachusetts	22.5	South Dakota	34.3
Rhode Island	22.6	Arizona	34.4
New Jersey	23.1	Kansas	34.8
Connecticut	25.2	Nebraska	35.2
New Hampshire	25.5	Kentucky	35.4
Vermont	25.8	Louisiana	35.7
Maryland	26.6	Georgia	35.8
Maine	26.9	South Carolina	35.8
North Dakota	27.6	Alabama	35.9
Pennsylvania	27.7	Tennessee	36.0
Wisconsin	28.2	Missouri	36.9
Florida	28.2	North Carolina	36.9
Illinois	28.3	Mississippi	37.5
Minnesota	28.5	Nevada	37.8
Michigan	30.2	Colorado	38.1
Ohio	30.4	West Virginia	39.3
Delaware	31.2	Idaho	39.4
Virginia	31.3	Montana	40.0
Iowa	31.6	Texas	40.9
Utah	31.8	Arkansas	41.2
California	32.0	New Mexico	41.3
Hawaii	32.0	Oklahoma	41.7
Oregon	32.9	Wyoming	47.9
Indiana	33.6		

Table 2-5 The First Model for Cancer Deaths without Lung in 2010-2012. The Role of Higher Earth Magnetism (roughly more north)(more deaths) and More Rain (more deaths).

Model Summary

Model	R	R Square	Adjusted R Square	Std. Error of the Estimate
1	.940[a]	.883	.873	7.1661

a. Predictors: (Constant), DOGHOUSE, GEOMAG08, AGE65IN6, RAIN2

Coefficients[a]

Model		Unstandardized Coefficients		Standardized Coefficients	t	Sig.
		B	Std. Error	Beta		
1	(Constant)	-69.294	20.712		-3.346	.002
	AGE65IN6	10.088	.647	.840	15.596	.000
	GEOMAG08	1.738E-03	.000	.288	5.593	.000
	RAIN2	.403	.076	.286	5.274	.000
	DOGHOUSE	.507	.156	.172	3.260	.002

a. Dependent Variable: CANOLUNG

Correlations

		AGE65IN6	GEOMAG08	RAIN2	DOGHOUSE	CANOLUNG
AGE65IN6	Pearson Correlation	1	-.144	.305*	-.175	.856**
	Sig. (2-tailed)	.	.315	.029	.220	.000
	N	51	51	51	51	51
GEOMAG08	Pearson Correlation	-.144	1	-.074	-.086	.131
	Sig. (2-tailed)	.315	.	.604	.549	.359
	N	51	51	51	51	51
RAIN2	Pearson Correlation	.305*	-.074	1	-.237	.480**
	Sig. (2-tailed)	.029	.604	.	.095	.000
	N	51	51	51	51	51
DOGHOUSE	Pearson Correlation	-.175	-.086	-.237	1	-.067
	Sig. (2-tailed)	.220	.549	.095	.	.638
	N	51	51	51	51	51
CANOLUNG	Pearson Correlation	.856**	.131	.480**	-.067	1
	Sig. (2-tailed)	.000	.359	.000	.638	.
	N	51	51	51	51	51

*. Correlation is significant at the 0.05 level (2-tailed).
**. Correlation is significant at the 0.01 level (2-tailed).

Now, we can begin looking over the main model page for cancer minus lung in Table 2-5. Beginning in the last box, on the second page of this table, we check to make sure the correlation between the items in the model are reasonably low as a way to ensure validity. None are linked on the level of two stars, a good thing, but one is connected with one star, at the .05 level. There is a connection between age and rain (+.305*), not great but not bad either given the low size of the correlation.

As an extra, in the bottom row, repeated in the right row, is the link between each item and what we are examining, deaths from cancer without lung. We learn there are two significant items (with two stars), a link between older age and cancer, as well as a link between rain and cancer. There is no "zero order correlation" linking the other two items to cancer - between geomagnetism and cancer, and between having a dog and cancer. For these, we need the full model for the link to become clear. Only after accounting for the other items do these connections with cancer become apparent.

Now we can move on to the main model also in Table 2-5, the first two boxes. Looking at the top box, Adjusted R Square, we see that the model accounts for .873 or 87.3% of the total pattern (of variation between states in death rates from cancer without lung).

Now to the middle box, we first look at statistical significance to gain confidence that the results are "solid". Starting on the right, Sig. (t) is all below .01, all .000 except for dog which is .002, not perfect but still well below .01, suggesting that the odds are less than one in a hundred that the connection between dog and cancer in this particular sample would not be present in the broader population of deaths from cancer in other years, or in other parts of the world (perhaps). Moving to the second column from the right "t", we see why the Sig. (t) is so low: a high t score which should be over 2. These are all way over, from 3 to more than 15 (for age). Solid.

Next is the Beta column where we see the size order of each effect. In terms of size, these numbers can be compared directly to each other after ignoring the direction signs. The effects on cancer of geomagnetism and rain are almost exactly equal in size. Compared with having a dog, geomagnetism is a larger effect by 172/100=288/x. 28800=172x. 28800/172=x. 167.44=x. The effect on cancer of geomagnetism is about 67% larger, or some two thirds larger than the effect of having a dog (literally households with a dog).

As for the impact of each effect on the total, first is the portion of each item that is responsible for the success of the part of the pattern we have explained. We add the Beta column ignoring the decimal points and signs for ease (840+288+286+172)=1586 and divide each number by the sum. 840/1586=53.0. Thus age accounts for 53% of the "variance explained", the part of the pattern we have captured in this model. 288/1586=.1816. Geomagnetism accounts for 18.2 percent of the pattern the model is able to explain. 286/1586=18. Rain accounts for 18 percent of the pattern of cancer deaths between states, and, lastly, 172/1586=10.8. Households with a dog accounts for about 11 percent of the cancer pattern between states that we were able to figure out.

Next, we desire to know the actual size of each effect in explaining the TOTAL effect of the pattern including the small portion we were unable to figure out. This is 100% minus the 87.3% we did figure out which includes that remaining 12.7 percent portion. To do this, we take the sum of the Beta values, and ask what that number would be for one hundred percent of the explanation. 1586/87.3=x/100. 87.3x=158600. x=158600/87.3. x=1816.7. Using this answer, we now divide each Beta value by this number to get the actual size of the total explanation which can be attributed to each item.

First is age: 840/1816.7=46.2 percent of the total pattern of cancer deaths across states. Geomagnetism is 288/1816.7=15.9 percent of the total pattern linked with geomagnetism or around 16 percent. Rain is 286/1816.7=15.7 percent of the total pattern, very close to that of geomagnetism. Lastly is households with a dog 172/1816.7=9.5%. Having a dog explains 9.5 percent of the total pattern of cancer deaths without lung across the states of the US.

The B column is the actual equation that summarizes the pattern of cancer deaths represented by all the 51 numbers (cancer death rates) in the list. The number for geomagnetism is 1.73E-03, which for purposes of manipulating the equation, can be rewritten by moving the decimal three places to the left or .001738.

Using this equation, we can now construct the most meaningful view of the pattern of dying from cancer without lung. We now "zero out" two of the items, age 65 and having a dog. We accomplish this zeroing out process by substituting the mean (average) value for all the cases instead of the actual value for each state, the percent age 65, and the percent of households with a dog. For the remaining two items, which will now be our focus, geomagnetism and rain, both linked with more deaths from cancer, we will use the actual value for each state.

We can do this now in the equation below. In SPSS version 11.0, we use the pull down menu in the data file "transform" and then "compute". We will name this list cmagrain for cancer magnetism rain (8 letter maximum).

We start by finding the means for the two items we wish to hold constant, to zero out: age and dog. In SPSS 11, that is in the data file, pull down menu analyze, then descriptive statistics, then descriptives, choosing items age65 and doghouse. The mean for age [age65in6] is 12.653, for households with a dog [doghouse] 32.406. In the equation, instead of adding the item name, we substitute these mean numbers thus knocking out the effect of the change in these items by state.

For the remaining two items we wish to vary, interested to know the impact of the change in these more interesting items: geomagnetism and rain, we put in the item name thus allowing these items to vary to see their impact.

We will do this now below using the equation from Table 2-5, second big box down, the B column. We do this back in the data file from the pull down menu choosing transform, compute, typing the name of the new list that we decided earlier to call cmagrain. The equation is (minus) -.69.294 + (10.088 * 12.653) +(.001738 * geomag08) + (.403 * rain2) + (.507 * 32.406).

Looking now at Table 2-6 Cmagrain, the result of this endeavor, we have the best view yet of the pattern of cancer death rates without lung. To repeat, this view zeroes out the effects of older age and having a dog (both "bad", meaning linked with more deaths) and helps us to see how the pattern is affected by the two environmental patterns of interest: geomagnetism and rain, both bad as well, it so happens.

Table 2-6 cmagrain (cancer without lung magnetism rain).

Most meaningful view of cancer death rates without lung in 2010-2012: the negative role of Earth magnetism and rain. Setting aside the impact of older age as well as households with dogs by holding them constant. Varying geomagnetism (more deaths) and rain (more deaths).

Hawaii	144.82	Georgia	182.80
Arizona	162.22	Pennsylvania	182.83
Nevada	162.55	Missouri	182.93
California	163.71	Virginia	182.99
New Mexico	165.71	Michigan	183.07
North Dakota	171.00	Alabama	183.10
Idaho	172.81	Iowa	183.40
Utah	172.92	West Virginia	183.42
Colorado	173.41	Mississippi	183.59
Wyoming	174.19	Massachusetts	183.64
Florida	175.66	Ohio	183.66
Montana	176.14	Louisiana	183.71
Oklahoma	177.64	Minnesota	184.03
Alaska	178.30	New Jersey	184.25
Kansas	179.57	Arkansas	184.30
North Carolina	179.85	Wisconsin	184.32
Texas	180.08	Indiana	184.33
Nebraska	181.28	Connecticut	184.40
District	181.28	Illinois	184.49
South Dakota	181.42	Kentucky	184.60
Delaware	181.99	Washington	184.61
Oregon	182.31	Rhode Island	184.91
New Hampshire	182.35	Tennessee	185.13
Maryland	182.43	New York	185.46
Vermont	182.70	Maine	185.84
South Carolina	182.78		

Americans can all see where their own state falls on Table 2-6. Hawaii is best with the lowest death rate. The dry, low-rain states of the US southwest also do very well. Poor Rhode Island and New York do badly for this cancer without lung with New York second to last at number 50 best (out of 51).

Florida is number 11 best. While Florida is "bad" for rain, it has low geomagnetism being the second lowest state for that. Returning to number 1 Hawaii, I would just like to comment that not only is its geomagnetism lowest (best) but, despite being "tropical", it also has relatively little rain, at least in Honolulu, the biggest city, where there is 22 inches of rain over the course of the year.

Now is the time for some brief commentary on the results here. For this, we can return to the main model in Table 2-5 called canolung, cancer without lung. These numbers in the B column are the numerical summary of the model in the form of an equation which was an attempt to explain the original pattern of deaths across all of the states (in Table 2-1).

Once again in this cancer model without lung, older age comes out as a huge item helping to explain the pattern between states. To repeat my thinking from the previous model of all cancer deaths, dying in general is linked with older age as is dying from cancer in particular. This is not true for every single disease from which people die but it is generally true. In this and all other cancer models, it was necessary to test for the effect of older age because it usually proves to be connected and must be considered for inclusion in the model as a control before we can look at other connections that might be less well known.

The finding about stronger geomagnetism on the ground being linked with more deaths from cancer is perhaps the most important new result of the model. This finding only becomes apparent once lung cancer is removed and we had a chance to look at other cancers, still the large majority (as lung accounts for about 28 percent of all deaths from cancer). It is quite a mystery why higher magnetism whose origin is inside the Earth might help to explain the pattern of cancer deaths.

Rain comes out once again as an item in this model linked with deaths from cancer, even without lung cancer included here. To repeat from the last chapter, rain signals to me a role for bacteria in the development of cancer as increased bacterial growth generally goes together with an increase in moisture, a necessary condition for such growth. Two additional ideas are an increase in gamma radiation from rain and thunderstorms, as well as a decrease in body voltage, body electricity in the period before, during, and after rain (based on my own experimenting with a body voltage meter).

Having a dog might be linked with more deaths from cancer, probably a first finding, however disconcerting, establishing such a link on a macro statistical level. In this model, the more households with dogs, the more deaths from cancer in a state. I should note that this research does not establish the more micro finding comparing households with and without a dog and showing cancer deaths higher in the former. Rather, this is on a state level. The more households with a dog in a state, the more deaths from cancer in that state (per hundred thousand people).

We do not know for sure if this is the case because people from those dog households are the ones responsible for the higher cancer death rate, more likely to die from cancer. Furthermore, it is possible that even if people living with dogs were more likely to die of these cancers, it might be due to some characteristic they have in common that has nothing directly to do with living with a dog per se. While nothing is certain, it seems easiest to assume that it is people with the dogs who are more likely to die from these cancers and that it is possible that this is due, sadly, to their interaction with their dogs.

Lastly, we can compare the two cancer models to each other, the one for all deaths from cancer in Chapter 1 to this model of deaths from cancer minus lung cancer here in Chapter 2. In so doing, we must mention items that did not make it into the second model without lung.

The first of these is smokers. In the first model of all deaths from cancer (including lung), this item clearly provided evidence for the link between smoking and cancer. I was thankful for it, in light of so many new findings in this research. At least that well-established link appeared. In this second model of cancer deaths without lung, the smoking item does not appear! This suggests that smoking is linked to cancer because of lung cancer and without lung cancer, smoking does not explain deaths from all other kinds of cancer (together) in a way that can be discerned statistically.

To put this null finding in perspective, two comments are in order. First, it is still possible that smoking might be an influence in cancer deaths of specific kinds. We would only know whether or not such was the case by doing separate models for each kind of cancer (which happen to follow in subsequent chapters for many cancers). All we are able to say is that, after excluding lung cancer, smoking is not significantly related to all deaths from the cancers that remain as a group, overall.

Second, a null finding does not mean that smoking has no harmful effect. Rather, it suggests that whatever harmful effect there might be on cancer in general without lung, it is not strong enough to make it into this final model, strong enough to be identified by this statistical method as related. Generally speaking, only very large items can be identified with this method and smoking does not appear to have made the cut (once lung cancer is removed).

Lastly is the unusual finding about Jews being linked to fewer deaths from cancer in the full cancer model of Chapter 1. It is still possible to build this model with Jews. In a model not shown, Jews is still linked with fewer deaths from cancer less lung. In a decision on my part, I decided to replace the item about percent Jews with the item about households with dogs.

Around this question, I did some additional "testing" beyond these final models to help clarify some complicated connections. In a model without dog and with Jews, the explanatory power of the model increases from .873 to .879. The introduction of Jews knocks out dogs from the model but I have decided to go with the final model with dogs in the hope that it might be more illuminating for learning about cancer.

Regardless, Jews and dogs are unable to be together in the model because of their high correlation of minus -.645. The more Jews in a state, the fewer the households with dogs. Furthermore, they weaken each other in the same model with both becoming not significant. This suggests that part of the reason why Jews might be less likely to die from cancer without lung is because they are less likely to live in households with a dog, assuming that dogs are somehow linked with cancer.

Furthermore, thinking about the main finding in the full cancer model in Chapter 1, dogs might be the reason why Jews are less likely to die of cancer of all kinds. I will double check this new idea now by redoing the main model of all cancer deaths (from Chapter 1) with dogs added. In this model for cancer for all kinds in 2010-2012, dog does weaken Jews to a level of marginal signficance (Sig. t .010) suggesting, that one part of the explanation for why Jews might be less likely to die from cancer is because they are less likely to live in households with a dog. I should note, however, that this experimental model is merely a test because the high correlation between dogs and Jews in a negative direction makes it a violation of the rules of regression having both in the same model at one time.

After this additional testing, I am now persuaded of two things. First, having a dog might well be connected with dying from cancer excluding cancer of the lungs. Second, the connection between having a dog and cancer works rather well for explaining why Jews might be less likely to die from cancer. They are less likely to live in households in which there is a dog present.

In a final additional model, I returned to the all cancer deaths model in Chapter 1 and tested the dog item in that model. Adding the dog item without Jews yields a marginally significant result of Sig. t .009, too weak for my standards. It did vaguely affirm, however, that even with lung cancer included, having a dog might be linked with cancer. So the introduction of the dog matter helps explain cancer as well as the finding linking Jews with fewer deaths from cancer.

Chapter 3. Dying from lung cancer - a link with insufficiently strong ultraviolet in sunlight where people live?

As we already know from the last chapter, lung cancer is the biggest cancer. Death rates from this disease account for 27.7 percent of all deaths in the cancer death rate category, over a quarter. In terms of individual deaths, a 2015 estimate of deaths from lung cancer is 158,040 in the United States. In this research, when I speak of lung cancer, I am referring to the larger death category called "[m]alignant neoplasms of trachea, bronchus and lung" and it includes those deaths as well.

We begin with Table 3-1, as usual, a yearly average based on a three year period, in this case, death rates from lung cancer for the years 2011, 2012 and 2013. Utah has the lowest death rate at about 23 deaths per hundred thousand people and Kentucky has the highest death rate at about 103 deaths. The mean (average) value is 68.0 deaths (rounded).

Building a model for lung cancer was a somewhat unusual endeavor because many of the items with which the pattern between states is connected also happen to be correlated with each other. This violates the rules of the method raising questions about the validity of the results. On the other hand, it makes it possible to build a variety of models.

Some examples of this situation follow: items linked with lung cancer but also with other items. Percent age 65 (more deaths from lung cancer) is linked with going to college (fewer deaths from lung cancer). This correlation between older age and going to college is in a negative direction (-.501). More older people in the population, fewer people who attended college. Another example is with smoking (more deaths from lung cancer). Attending college is associated in a negative direction with smoking every day (-.668).

In the latter models, (lung cancer being among the last even though I place this research as Chapter 3), I tightened up on my willingness to tolerate these intercorrelations between items in an attempt to improve the validity of the final model. This has, generally speaking, resulted in a shorter model with fewer items, but one whose conclusions are more solid with less concern that the result might come from any strange effect from the connectedness between the items in the model.

Table 3-1 lung1113.

Lung cancer death rate between 2011 and 2013, yearly average (per hundred thousand people), by state.

State	Rate	State	Rate
Utah	22.5	Wisconsin	67.9
Colorado	39.9	Kansas	68.8
California	43.7	South Dakota	69.3
New Mexico	46.8	Vermont	71.2
District	46.9	New Hampshire	71.4
Hawaii	49.0	North Carolina	73.7
Alaska	49.1	Iowa	74.9
Texas	50.4	Rhode Island	75.6
Wyoming	52.0	Pennsylvania	76.3
Idaho	53.2	Michigan	76.5
Arizona	55.8	South Carolina	77.6
Minnesota	57.2	Florida	77.8
Washington	58.2	Louisiana	78.1
New Jersey	59.4	Delaware	79.1
Maryland	59.6	Indiana	80.0
New York	59.6	Ohio	83.3
Connecticut	60.3	Alabama	84.7
Georgia	61.6	Missouri	85.3
North Dakota	62.4	Oklahoma	85.4
Virginia	62.7	Mississippi	86.5
Nevada	63.2	Tennessee	87.4
Nebraska	64.3	Maine	91.1
Massachusetts	64.9	Arkansas	95.5
Montana	66.8	West Virginia	100.2
Illinois	67.4	Kentucky	103.4
Oregon	67.7		

In making these decisions, I tried to follow standard rules such as reducing multicollinearity (intercorrelation between items). There is probably a small role played by my personal judgment as well. Due to this problem of intercorrelation, I decided for the final model to use "college" to represent both older age and smoking with which it is connected (in a negative direction).

The final lung cancer model is in Table 3-4. It consists of two items. The first is attending college. The more people in the state who attended college, the fewer the deaths from lung cancer. The second item is ultraviolet, based on the intensity of ultraviolet reaching the ground around noon time as captured in the NOAA UVI (Ultraviolet Index) over a nine year period in the largest city of the state. The stronger the ultraviolet in sunlight reaching the ground in that city over the course of many years, the fewer the deaths from lung cancer.

As in previous chapters, I include the actual lists for each item in the model with the values for each state. Table 3-2 is the list by state for attending college. These attenders include people who attended even for a short time up to those who graduated with a degree. The lowest state is West Virginia where around 29 percent attended college. The highest is Colorado where around 58 percent have attended college. The average (mean) of all the states (including "District" which stands for District of Columbia or Washington DC) is about 45 percent.

The second item in the model is ultraviolet [uvi0614] using the UV Index between 2006 and 2014. This is based on the UV Index estimates from NOAA kindly constructed by Craig Long for this long period of time, nine years. This average UV Index value for each state is actually the value for the largest city in that state over this period of years. This is a sophisticated model-based estimate of the amount of ultraviolet reaching the ground in that city at "solar noon" when the sun is at its peak overhead and includes predicted cloudiness and other weather conditions that would affect the intensity of this part of sunlight that might reach the ground. I cannot express too often my feeling of gratitude for the cooperation of Mr. Long from NOAA in creating this aggregation of UV Index values for this extended period. Of course, the results of this research are not endorsed in any way by Mr. Long or NOAA.

This nine year average of the intensity of ultraviolet reaching the ground for the largest city in each state can be found in Table 3-3. The low is in Alaska with a UVI (UV Index) of around 2 while the high is in Hawaii with a UVI of around 11. The mean UVI for all the states is around 5.

Table 3-2 sumcolig some college.

Percent of the population in a state who have attended college (without necessarily having gotten a degree).

State	%	State	%
West Virginia	29.3	Illinois	46.3
Kentucky	32.9	Texas	46.7
Arkansas	33.7	Nebraska	47.2
Pennsylvania	36.0	Nevada	47.3
Louisiana	36.6	Montana	47.5
Mississippi	36.9	Kansas	48.4
Tennessee	37.0	South Dakota	48.4
Alabama	37.4	North Dakota	48.5
Indiana	37.5	Virginia	48.5
South Carolina	38.7	Idaho	49.4
Ohio	39.3	Minnesota	49.5
Missouri	40.7	Connecticut	49.7
North Carolina	41.0	Wyoming	49.9
Georgia	41.3	Massachusetts	50.2
Wisconsin	41.5	Maryland	50.3
Iowa	41.6	New Hampshire	50.4
Maine	41.8	Hawaii	51.3
Rhode Island	42.6	District	52.0
Oklahoma	44.1	Arizona	52.5
Florida	44.3	Oregon	52.5
Michigan	44.4	California	53.9
Delaware	44.8	Washington	55.8
New York	45.3	Alaska	57.8
New Jersey	45.5	Utah	57.9
Vermont	46.2	Colorado	57.9
New Mexico	46.3		

Table 3-3 uvi0614.ultraviolet.
Average annual UVI (UV Index) score in the largest city of the state over a nine year period between 2006 and 2014.

State	UVI	State	UVI
Alaska	1.9	District	4.6
Washington	3.5	Kentucky	4.8
Vermont	3.6	Missouri	4.8
Oregon	3.6	Idaho	4.9
Maine	3.9	Kansas	5.2
North Dakota	3.9	North Carolina	5.4
Minnesota	3.9	Virginia	5.4
Michigan	4.0	Tennessee	5.5
New Hampshire	4.0	Wyoming	5.5
Wisconsin	4.1	Arkansas	5.6
Ohio	4.2	Oklahoma	5.6
Rhode Island	4.2	Utah	5.7
Illinois	4.2	Colorado	5.8
South Dakota	4.2	Georgia	6.0
Connecticut	4.2	South Carolina	6.3
Massachusetts	4.2	Nevada	6.3
Iowa	4.3	Mississippi	6.4
Pennsylvania	4.4	Texas	6.9
New York	4.4	Arizona	6.9
Montana	4.4	Alabama	7.0
Indiana	4.5	New Mexico	7.0
Nebraska	4.5	California	7.0
West Virginia	4.6	Louisiana	7.2
Delaware	4.6	Florida	8.5
New Jersey	4.6	Hawaii	11.1
Maryland	4.6		

Now we are ready to look at the final model in more detail found in Table 3-4. The model explains 75.7 percent of the pattern between all of the states. (In the top box, the Adjusted R Square is .757). The bottom box shows that the degree of correlation between both items is very low, a good thing. College and Ultraviolet are correlated hardly at all (-.080, not significant). The bottom line, showing lung deaths, reveals a strong negative correlation between college and lung cancer (-.853), more college, fewer deaths. There is no significant correlation between ultraviolet and lung deaths (-.128). Apparently, we have to first wait for the large impact of college on lung cancer deaths to be accounted for before that connection is able to reveal itself.

Having looked at correlations to gain assurance about the validity of the final model, we can now move to the middle box which includes the final model and basic information about it. Starting with statistical significance on the right, the connection between college and fewer deaths from lung cancer is very solid, (Sig. t .000, t over 12). The link between ultraviolet and fewer lung cancer deaths is also satisfactory in that it is under a Sig. value of .01 at .007 with a t value of about 2.8, needing to be above 2. (The stringent .01 level of significance is the standard for all the models in this book). I note that while the Sig. T value of .007 is satisfactory, it is not a perfect result.

Next, we look at the Beta column in the middle to evaluate the size of each effect, primarily in the context of the other. Together, both items add to 1.066 (ignoring the signs, .869+.197). Of the portion the model explains, college accounts for 81.5 percent of the total (.869/1.066), a huge amount. Ultraviolet accounts for the balance 18.5 percent of that total.

Because the model does not explain one hundred percent of the pattern but only some 76 percent, it is useful to know how much each explains of that total possible explanation. 1.066/.757=x/1. .757x=1.066. x=1.066/.757. x=1.408. This is the equivalent value for the entire pattern explained. For college, .869/1.408=.617. Of the total possible explanation of the pattern of lung cancer deaths between all of the states, attending college explains 61.7 percent. For ultraviolet, it is .197/1.408=.140. As a portion of the total possible explanation for lung cancer deaths as revealed in this

Table 3-4 The Lung Cancer Model: The Role of Not Strong Enough Ultraviolet in Sunlight (more deaths).

Model Summary

Model	R	R Square	Adjusted R Square	Std. Error of the Estimate
1	.876[a]	.767	.757	7.9234

a. Predictors: (Constant), UVI0614, SUMCOLIG

Coefficients[a]

Model		Unstandardized Coefficients		Standardized Coefficients	t	Sig.
		B	Std. Error	Beta		
1	(Constant)	174.371	8.954		19.473	.000
	SUMCOLIG	-2.103	.169	-.869	-12.419	.000
	UVI0614	-2.126	.756	-.197	-2.813	.007

a. Dependent Variable: LUNG1113

Correlations

		SUMCOLIG	UVI0614	LUNG1113
SUMCOLIG	Pearson Correlation	1	-.080	-.853**
	Sig. (2-tailed)	.	.578	.000
	N	51	51	51
UVI0614	Pearson Correlation	-.080	1	-.128
	Sig. (2-tailed)	.578	.	.372
	N	51	51	51
LUNG1113	Pearson Correlation	-.853**	-.128	1
	Sig. (2-tailed)	.000	.372	.
	N	51	51	51

**. Correlation is significant at the 0.01 level (2-tailed).

"state by state" list, ultraviolet explains .140, or 14 percent. After accounting for the large impact of attending college on the pattern of dying from lung cancer (fewer deaths), ultraviolet reaching the ground accounts for 14 percent of that total pattern. The stronger the intensity of ultraviolet in sunlight that reaches the ground, the fewer the deaths from lung cancer in that state.

Now we can use the B column in the middle box of Table 3-4, which contains the actual equation of the final lung cancer model, to calculate what we consider a new list of states, our choice of a "best view". The huge connection between not going to college and dying from lung cancer will be discussed afterwards. Since our primary focus in this research is on environmental factors, it is most interesting now to try and understand this effect on lung cancer of ultraviolet in sunlight.

There is a way of looking at this effect of ultraviolet on lung cancer after holding to the side the large impact of the demographic item of college (being one way that some people are different from others). We can create this "best view" by holding constant the effect of college by using its mean (average value of all the states) instead of the actual value for each state. By using the original equation from the B column and plugging in this average value for college, we can get a better view of the effect of ultraviolet on the story of dying from lung cancer in the United States.

The equation for constructing this "best view" from the B column is as follows. 174.371 - (2.103 times the college mean, 45.422) - (2.126 times the value of the UVI for each state in Table 3-3 [uvi0614]). I will do this now using transform, compute, from the data box in SPSS 11, called lunguvil, which stands for lung UVI list.

This "best view" lung cancer list can now be seen in Table 3-5 lunguvil. Based on the actual lung cancer death rates that appear in Table 3-1, this is what the list looks like after neutralizing the effect of college on that lung cancer death rate list. What remains, then, is the other item, ultraviolet and its effect. Of course, I should point out that the ordering of the states is exactly the same as the ultraviolet list in Table 3-3 but with the direction reversed. As ultraviolet is the only item allowed to "vary", the higher the ultraviolet score goes in Table 3-3, the lower the death rate from lung cancer in Table 3-5. In this "best view" of lung cancer death rates after accounting for whether people attended college, this is the predicted death rate from lung cancer showing the effect of ultraviolet on the rate.

Table 3-5 lunguvil. lung - UV Index list.
Best view of lung cancer death rates by state after setting aside the huge effect of college (fewer deaths). Predicted deaths (per hundred thousand) based on actual death rates in 2011-2013 but varying only insufficient ultraviolet reaching the ground (more deaths).

State	Rate	State	Rate
Hawaii	55.2	New Jersey	69.1
Florida	60.8	Maryland	69.1
Louisiana	63.5	District	69.1
Alabama	64.0	Indiana	69.3
New Mexico	64.0	Nebraska	69.3
California	64.0	Pennsylvania	69.5
Texas	64.2	New York	69.5
Arizona	64.2	Montana	69.5
Mississippi	65.2	Iowa	69.7
South Carolina	65.5	Ohio	69.9
Nevada	65.5	Rhode Island	69.9
Georgia	66.1	Illinois	69.9
Colorado	66.5	South Dakota	69.9
Utah	66.7	Connecticut	69.9
Arkansas	66.9	Massachusetts	69.9
Oklahoma	66.9	Wisconsin	70.1
Tennessee	67.2	Michigan	70.3
Wyoming	67.2	New Hampshire	70.3
North Carolina	67.4	Maine	70.6
Virginia	67.4	North Dakota	70.6
Kansas	67.8	Minnesota	70.6
Idaho	68.4	Vermont	71.2
Kentucky	68.6	Oregon	71.2
Missouri	68.6	Washington	71.4
West Virginia	69.1	Alaska	74.8
Delaware	69.1		

This predicted lung cancer death rate in Table 3-5 shows that Hawaii would have the lowest lung cancer death rate given that the sun is strongest there, 55.2 deaths per hundred thousand people. Highest is in Alaska given that it has the least strong "sun" of all the states in the ultraviolet list in Table 3-3, with the highest predicted death rate from lung cancer of 74.8 deaths.

Compared to the predicted rate in Hawaii, the predicted rate in Alaska is how much higher? 55.2/100=74.8/x. 55.2x=748. x=748/55.2. x=13.55. The predicted death rate from lung cancer attributable to differences in sun is about 13.6 percent higher in the state with the weakest sun (Alaska) compared to the state with the strongest sun (Hawaii).

This is another way, then, to assess the overall effect of the main finding in this model, the impact of insufficiently strong ultraviolet from sunlight on the death rate from lung cancer (more deaths). This result of 13.6 percent is very close to the previous assessment of the size of this effect where the conclusion was that "sun" explained 14 percent of the pattern between all the states in dying from the biggest cancer.

With the main environmental finding quantified, it is worth going back to the college connection (more people who have been to college, fewer death from lung cancer). To understand the large effect of college, we must return now to the link between college and both smoking and older age (age 65 plus) with which they are correlated in a negative direction (one up, the other down). None of these are able to be in the same model because of this intercorrelation. I chose college based on the standard rules suggesting that is the best choice.

The link between college and lung cancer is so strong partly because people who have been to college are less likely to smoke.

This huge effect of college is also partly due to the fact that the more people who have been to college, the fewer older people there are in that state over the age of 65 (as a percent of the population). As older people are more likely to die from cancer and to die in general, it makes sense that more college attenders in a state signals a younger population and thus, fewer deaths.

Nevertheless, because in a test with all three items, college still survives, being linked with lung cancer deaths, these two items of smoking and older age do not provide the entire explanation for why college is so strongly linked with fewer deaths from lung cancer. There is more to the story, part of the broader unanswered question of the strong impact that college has on reducing death rates.

While attending college might suggest membership in a higher social class, this still does not answer the question about why the powerful effect. I am at a loss to explain this effect even after years of pondering the question. Just to repeat, the large effect of college on lung cancer death rates goes beyond any difference in smoking cigarettes between those who did and did not attend college.

Ultraviolet reaching the ground is what I call a "north south" item. We all know that the sun gets weaker as we travel from the south in the United States to the north. This is true regardless of the season if we drive on the East Coast, from say Key West Florida, and go north on Interstate 95, to say Portland Maine. It has something to do with the tilt of the Earth away from the sun the farther from the equator we are. The strength of sunlight, of which ultraviolet is part, then, is, obviously one of those things that varies primarily from south to north.

There are many other such environmental differences about which we are also very familiar. One example is average temperature. As we go north in the United States, it gets colder when considering the entire year, generally speaking.

Why, then, did I pick ultraviolet rather than other "north south" items? While the answer is obvious to me, I wanted to state it explicitly for fear it might not be as obvious to others. I tested ultraviolet against other "north south" items and it worked better, was more strongly linked with the pattern of deaths from lung cancer than the other ones.

While typically tested at the time I am building the model, I added three additional "north south" items as an extra test. They are average air temperature over the course of the year in each city (one city per state), the strength of geomagnetism measured on the ground in the city which gets stronger as we move north. The third was total solar energy reaching the ground over the year in the city, another measure of sunlight but different than the one exclusively measuring ultraviolet (among other differences as well). These other items do not stand up, get easily eliminated, leaving ultraviolet as the winner. So I picked ultraviolet because it happened to be the "north south" item that linked up best with the pattern of deaths from lung cancer using the state death rates in Table 3-1.

Now comes the time to think about the main finding of the lung cancer model - a connection to insufficiently strong ultraviolet in sunlight.

I wish to first raise the unlikely possibility that the finding has nothing to do with human exposure to ultraviolet per se. Perhaps the intensity of ultraviolet has an effect on the environment in some unspecified way that, in turn, affects how many people die from lung cancer. While this is possible, I am unable to identify what this indirect effect might be and therefore, find it unlikely and unsatisfying as an explanation for the main finding here.

Second, I should note the weakness of the finding because the UV Index is no direct measure of exposure to sunlight at all. It is the ultimate "macro" measure using satellite data from way up above the Earth to help construct this estimate of ultraviolet reaching the ground in each location. Ultraviolet is highest around noon (solar noon when the ultraviolet portion is highest of the entire day). This varies by place and time of year because each city is in a different location within the time zone band. Also, daylight savings time moves the clock one hour forward thus also moving the time of solar noon. (I think all the states move the clocks except Hawaii). While close to impossible in such a macro study, measuring actual exposure of people to sunlight around noon would be a great challenge in any study.

Furthermore, I do not know whether or not being outside and exposure to noon time sun varies from place to place. While we might assume that people are outside more in places with nicer weather, given that people typically work during the day in offices, it would be difficult to pin any interpretation of these results on this supposition. My guess is that exposure to sunlight around noon might not vary from place to place as much as we think with air conditioning playing a role in sun avoidance as office people might remain cocooned inside during lunch when it is hot out.

While adding considerable conjecture, my best interpretation is that the finding does have to do with direct exposure to sunlight. But if this might not vary from place to place, then what would explain the difference in death rates from lung cancer? It must be differences in the strength of the sun itself, which goes with its ultraviolet portion. A person living in a northern place such as Portland Maine or Seattle Washington might be outside at the "right" time of day when the ultraviolet is strongest. If the ultraviolet reaching the ground is not intense enough to do its posited cancer fighting job, however, it might not matter that much.

The most reasonable explanation for this link between insufficiently strong ultraviolet reaching the ground and more deaths from lung cancer is as follows. Exposure to the sun helps to prevent lung cancer but that this exposure must be to a sun that has a sufficiently strong intensity of ultraviolet to do its posited cancer fighting job.

As for what happens inside the body to make exposure to ultraviolet reduce the incidence of lung cancer deaths, I do not know. My best guess is that such exposure speeds up the cell cycle resulting in cell copies with fewer errors and hence, fewer cells that become cancerous.

This posited anti-cancer effect of ultraviolet in sunlight appears to conflict sharply with accepted views that this same ultraviolet is a cause of another kind of cancer, skin cancer. A future chapter here looks at death rates from the common skin cancer that causes people to die, melanoma. Assuming the conventional belief about ultraviolet as a major cause of melanoma for the moment, I wish to make the obvious modest point that lung cancer is responsible for far more deaths than skin cancer. In a given year, roughly 12,000 people die from skin cancer (in the United States) whereas 158,000 die from lung cancer, a number that is over 13 times larger.

Chapter 4. Breast cancer and a Link with Particle Air Pollution

My mother's mother died from breast cancer at around age 47 when my mother was only 12 years old. Of course, I never had a chance to meet the woman whom I hear had a beautiful singing voice. In the 2011-2013 set of years, the death rate from breast cancer is 17.2 deaths per hundred thousand. As with all the death rates, it is the category 18+ crude, meaning it is all the deaths from that disease in people age 18 and over divided by all the people in the state in that age group, age 18 and over (I think).

For all kinds of cancer, the US death rate is 241.4 deaths. The death rate from all causes is 1047.0. From these numbers, we learn first that, as a percent of all cancers, breast is (17.2/241.4) 7.1 percent of all deaths from cancer. As a percent of all the deaths recorded that year in death rate form, breast cancer is 17.2/1047.0 or 1.6 percent of all deaths. While some men die of breast cancer as well, of 100 deaths, 99 are women.

The breast cancer death rate list by state can be found in Table 4-1 Breast: Death Rate from breast cancer by state in 2011-2013 (per hundred thousand people). The lowest death rate is in Alaska with about 11 deaths (per hundred thousand). The highest death rate state for breast cancer is Pennsylvania with about 20 deaths per population size. This means that the rate in the lowest state is only about 53 percent the size of the rate in the highest state, about 47 percent lower.

That is a sizeable spread and I suspect it might be partly accounted for by environmental factors, the ways that the environment is different across the large country of the United States. It is our job now to find out what they might be in order to understand this disease a little better. However we may be interested in figuring out the cause, we are unable to prove it definitively due to the limitations of this particular scientific method. Unfortunately, all methods have both strengths and weaknesses.

There are only two items in the breast cancer model and let us begin by becoming familiar with the state lists for each item.

Table 4-2 is Particle Pollution [PM07]: Fine particle air pollution, particulate matter 2.5 microns in the largest city of the state averaged over the year 2007.

Table 4-1 Breast:
Death rate from breast cancer by state in 2011-2013
(per hundred thousand people)

State	Rate	State	Rate
Alaska	10.9	Montana	17.4
Hawaii	11.9	North Carolina	17.4
Utah	12.8	New York	17.5
Colorado	14.1	Wisconsin	17.7
Texas	14.5	Indiana	18.0
North Dakota	14.8	Maryland	18.1
Wyoming	14.9	Alabama	18.2
New Mexico	15.0	South Dakota	18.3
Washington	15.3	Tennessee	18.4
California	15.3	Kentucky	18.4
Idaho	15.6	Illinois	18.5
Minnesota	15.6	Florida	18.6
Arizona	15.9	Arkansas	18.6
Vermont	16.3	Delaware	18.6
Maine	16.4	South Carolina	18.7
Georgia	16.4	Michigan	18.8
Nevada	16.5	Oklahoma	18.9
New Hampshire	16.5	Louisiana	19.1
Massachusetts	16.5	Mississippi	19.1
Nebraska	16.8	Missouri	19.1
Oregon	16.9	District	19.5
Kansas	16.9	New Jersey	20.0
Virginia	16.9	West Virginia	20.1
Rhode Island	17.0	Ohio	20.2
Connecticut	17.2	Pennsylvania	20.4
Iowa	17.3		

Table 4-2 Particle Pollution [PM07]:
Fine particle air pollution, particulate matter 2.5 microns in the largest city of the state averaged over the year 2007

State	Value	State	Value
Hawaii	3.8	Utah	12.5
Wyoming	4.3	Mississippi	12.8
Alaska	4.6	Arkansas	12.9
New Mexico	6.7	Texas	13.0
Oregon	6.8	Tennessee	13.4
North Dakota	7.5	New Jersey	13.6
Montana	7.9	North Carolina	13.9
Washington	8.8	Michigan	14.0
Nebraska	9.0	Virginia	14.2
Vermont	9.3	District	14.3
Arizona	9.4	South Carolina	14.5
Florida	9.4	Maryland	15.0
Nevada	9.8	Delaware	15.0
Idaho	9.9	West Virginia	15.5
Maine	9.9	California	15.7
South Dakota	9.9	Kentucky	15.7
Minnesota	10.2	Illinois	15.7
Rhode Island	10.5	Pennsylvania	15.9
Colorado	10.8	New York	16.2
New Hampshire	10.8	Wisconsin	16.3
Iowa	11.3	Ohio	16.5
Louisiana	11.5	Georgia	16.7
Oklahoma	11.7	Indiana	17.0
Massachusetts	11.9	Missouri	17.3
Kansas	11.9	Alabama	20.6
Connecticut	12.1		

Particle pollution and ozone are the two most common air pollutants measured by the federal government in many locations across the country. Actually, it is done in cooperation with each state's environmental agency. These readings can be found in real time on airnow.gov.

This yearly average was from a different data source, also available for numerous locations across the country, wherever there is a monitoring station. I chose one location that seemed most appropriate to represent the entire city but really, in so doing, to represent the entire state. While I made a few attempts to do this for different pollutants and different years, this one, [pm07] (particulate matter in 2007) was the most successful. It worked for breast cancer in the sense that the statistical test uncovered a connection.

A number of years ago, the government moved from 10 microns to measuring even smaller particles in the air only 2.5 microns in size. This is a more difficult hurdle to pass with this more recent cutoff of smaller particles no larger than 2.5 microns. These particles are actually "dirt" in the air made of carbon. They are so small that they cannot be seen with the naked eye and a microscope must be used for viewing them. Their smaller size makes them easier to penetrate deep into the lungs when we breathe.

In this study, I found a link between how much particle pollution is typically in the air in the largest city of the state and how many deaths there are from breast cancer. The more of this microscopic dirt in the air, on average, over the course of the entire year, the more deaths from breast cancer.

Two things are worth emphasizing. First is that much of the earlier work on the effect of air pollution had an emphasis on breathing, respiration. This can still be seen from the descriptions on government websites about air pollution. More recently, evidence has been mounting of the even more serious effect of air pollution on heart disease, as well as increasing deaths in general, around periods of high levels.

The work here could be the first to show a link between particle air pollution and deaths from breast cancer. Many would expect it more likely to be linked with lung cancer. My tests of this idea for lung showed no confirmation that such is the case.

The second point worth emphasizing is the unusual "macro" use of local air pollution data in the context of a national study based on the counterintuitive idea that the largest city in the state might be able to represent the level of air pollution in the entire state (keeping in mind the crassness of this leap). In so doing, I have here been able to show a link again, on a national level, despite the imperfections, between one kind of air pollution, particulate matter, and breast cancer deaths in a given year across the entire country (organized by state).

The second item in the breast cancer model is our, by now, very familiar item of older age, age 65 and over in the state, found in Table 4-3. The percent seniors in a state goes from a low of about 7 percent in chilly Alaska, to a high of about 17 percent in balmy Florida.

Unsurprisingly, older age is linked with more deaths from breast cancer in a state. As with deaths in general, older people are more likely to die, and this is true for cancer in particular. What we learn here is that the same is also true for breast cancer. We must note, however, that, of the two items, air pollution is actually more closely linked with breast cancer than age is. Whenever an item "beats out" age, such a powerful item in general, it is worth noting due to its general rarity. We will soon see this ahead in the next look at the breast cancer model itself.

In Table 4-4 which includes the breast cancer model, we start, as usual, with the correlations in the bottom box. The main purpose of this is to make sure there is no problem from connected items that might call into question the validity of the result. Looking at the first two lines, we see virtually no connection between particle pollution [PM07] and older age. I call this model "clean".

Next is the extra look at the zero order correlations with the matter at hand, breast cancer. While not essential when compared to examining the actual model, it can often be interesting. In this case, both particle pollution as well as age have connections with breast cancer on their own. There is a correlation of .628** between particle pollution and breast cancer. No minus sign means a plus direction. More particle pollution, more breast cancer. The same is true for age and breast cancer with its .563** correlation. More seniors, more deaths from breast cancer.

The top box shows the adjusted R square at .665, as this model explains 66.5 percent of the pattern between states. I decided to be satisfied with this simple model fearing to add African Americans which tends to be linked with breast cancer, more deaths. This was due to a random technical glitch related to the continuing geographic concentration of this population in the "old south", thus confounding tests of other geographic-linked items.

Table 4-3 Older age:
Percent age 65 and over in a state

State	%	State	%
Alaska	6.8	Oregon	12.9
Utah	8.8	Kansas	12.9
Georgia	9.8	New Jersey	12.9
Texas	9.9	Wisconsin	13.0
Colorado	10.0	New York	13.1
California	10.8	Oklahoma	13.2
Nevada	11.1	Nebraska	13.3
Washington	11.5	Vermont	13.3
Idaho	11.5	Massachusetts	13.3
Virginia	11.6	Missouri	13.3
Maryland	11.6	Connecticut	13.4
Illinois	12.0	Delaware	13.4
Minnesota	12.1	Ohio	13.4
Wyoming	12.2	Alabama	13.4
Louisiana	12.2	Montana	13.8
North Carolina	12.2	Rhode Island	13.9
District	12.3	Arkansas	13.9
New Mexico	12.4	Hawaii	14.0
New Hampshire	12.4	South Dakota	14.2
Mississippi	12.4	North Dakota	14.6
Indiana	12.4	Maine	14.6
Michigan	12.5	Iowa	14.6
Tennessee	12.7	Pennsylvania	15.2
Arizona	12.8	West Virginia	15.3
South Carolina	12.8	Florida	16.8
Kentucky	12.8		

Table 4-4 The Breast Cancer Model:
The Role of Particle Air Pollution (more deaths).

Model Summary

Model	R	R Square	Adjusted R Square	Std. Error of the Estimate
1	.824[a]	.678	.665	1.1900

a. Predictors: (Constant), AGE65IN6, PM07

Coefficients[a]

Model		Unstandardized Coefficients		Standardized Coefficients	t	Sig.
		B	Std. Error	Beta		
1	(Constant)	4.688	1.377		3.405	.001
	PM07	.340	.046	.602	7.340	.000
	AGE65IN6	.655	.101	.533	6.504	.000

a. Dependent Variable: BREST113

Correlations

		PM07	AGE65IN6	BREST113
PM07	Pearson Correlation	1	.050	.628**
	Sig. (2-tailed)	.	.728	.000
	N	51	51	51
AGE65IN6	Pearson Correlation	.050	1	.563**
	Sig. (2-tailed)	.728	.	.000
	N	51	51	51
BREST113	Pearson Correlation	.628**	.563**	1
	Sig. (2-tailed)	.000	.000	.
	N	51	51	51

**. Correlation is significant at the 0.01 level (2-tailed).

Now for the two item breast cancer model itself in Table 4-4. As usual, we start with statistical significance in the right most two boxes. Sig. is .000 with t values way over 2, particle pollution over 7 and age over 6, solid results.

Next is the size of the effect in the Beta column, both with plus signs (no minus sign) meaning positive in direction: more particle pollution, more breast cancer, and more older age population, more breast cancer deaths.

As already noted, particle pollution is larger than age and is listed first. Looking at the Beta column, we can begin to get a clearer view of the size of these effects on the pattern of breast cancer death rates. Without decimals, we add the two effects together (602+533=1135). Of the portion of the pattern that the model succeeds in explaining, particle pollution [pm07] accounts for 602/1135 or 53 percent. The portion of the pattern explained by older age [age65in6] is 533/1135 or about 47 percent.

Of the entire explanation, it would be less because the model only succeeds in explaining 66.5% of that total (the Adjusted R Square being .665). To find the actual portion of the total explanation for each item, we use algebra to get a new denominator. 1135/66.5=x/100. 66.5x=113500. x=113500/66.5. x=1706.77. We can now divide each Beta value by that number.

For particle pollution, it is 602/1706.77=35.27. Particle pollution accounts for about 35 percent of the total pattern of breast cancer death rates between the states. For older age, it is 533/1706.77=31.23. Older age accounts for about 31 percent of the total explanation of the breast cancer death pattern. Taken together, both items account for 66.5 percent of the pattern, the exact number of the Adjusted R Square.

This leaves 33.5 percent of the pattern that is NOT explained by the items in this model, a third. Overall, we learn that particle pollution accounts for a bit more than a third of the pattern, of the explanation, for why breast cancer death rates vary across states. Age accounts for a little less than a third of the pattern with the remaining third still open, unexplained in this work.

Next we move to the B column to use the equation itself for constructing a new list for breast cancer deaths that makes the most sense for purposes of learning. In this simple two items model, the decision here seems obvious. The link with older age is no surprise.

Continuing with my logic about the role of older age, it is likely (but not certain) that older age is linked with more breast cancer deaths because it is older people themselves who are doing the "extra" dying. For a younger person, however, it probably makes little difference if they move to a state with more older people because their chances of dying would probably not be affected.

This may even be the case for an older person whose chances of dying would probably also not be affected by how many older people happened to live in their state. (This could even reduce their chances of dying because there might be better hospitals, more experience in dealing with this disease. It is unlikely, however, that any such impact would be large enough to show up in a model such as this one – so macro (broad) in nature that only very large connections can pass the necessary tests). What we really want to view is the pattern of deaths AFTER accounting for this familiar effect of older age.

We do this by running the equation using the mean value instead of the actual state value for the percent seniors, age 65 and over. For the item whose effect we are interested to view, we use the actual state value. We can do that now using the equation numbers in the B column, from the data file in SPSS 11 pulling down the "transform" window and selecting "compute". We can call this list "brstdirt" for breast dirt, dirty air from particle air pollution.

The equation is as follows: brstdrt = 4.688 + (.340 * pm07) + (.655 * 12.653).

This new list can be found in Table 4-5 Brstdrt (Breast Dirt): The bad effect of fine particle air pollution on breast cancer death rates in 2011-2013 after accounting for the effect of older age (bad). Predicted death rates are for age 18 and over per hundred thousand people.

The state with the lowest predicted death rate is Hawaii with about 14 deaths. The highest predicted death rate from breast cancer is Alabama with about 20 deaths. This means that, compared with the highest death rate state, the rate in the lowest state is only 71 percent the size or lower by (100-71.42=28.58) about 29 percent. This is another way to see the size of this one item, small particle air pollution (2.5 microns) on deaths from breast cancer.

To make sure the point is obvious, because we are varying only the one item, particle air pollution, in Table 4-5, the ordering of the states in this predicted breast cancer list is identical to the ordering of the states in Table 4-2 Particle Polluution.

Table 4-5 Brstdrt (Breast Dirt):
The bad effect of fine particle air pollution on breast cancer death rates in 2011-2013 after accounting for the effect of older age (bad). Predicted death rates are for age 18 and over per hundred thousand people.

State	Rate	State	Rate
Hawaii	14.27	Utah	17.23
Wyoming	14.44	Mississippi	17.33
Alaska	14.54	Arkansas	17.36
New Mexico	15.25	Texas	17.40
Oregon	15.29	Tennessee	17.53
North Dakota	15.53	New Jersey	17.60
Montana	15.66	North Carolina	17.70
Washington	15.97	Michigan	17.74
Nebraska	16.04	Virginia	17.80
Vermont	16.14	District	17.84
Arizona	16.17	South Carolina	17.91
Florida	16.17	Maryland	18.08
Nevada	16.31	Delaware	18.08
Idaho	16.34	West Virginia	18.25
South Dakota	16.34	California	18.31
Maine	16.34	Illinois	18.31
Minnesota	16.44	Kentucky	18.31
Rhode Island	16.55	Pennsylvania	18.38
Colorado	16.65	New York	18.48
New Hampshire	16.65	Wisconsin	18.52
Iowa	16.82	Ohio	18.59
Louisiana	16.89	Georgia	18.65
Oklahoma	16.95	Indiana	18.76
Kansas	17.02	Missouri	18.86
Massachusetts	17.02	Alabama	19.98
Connecticut	17.09		

Now is the time for any additional thoughts I might have about the result. While I have nothing more to add about the link between older age and dying from breast cancer, the connection with particle air pollution strikes me as rather shocking in its clarity. What could possibly be the mechanism linking the two things together: dirt in the air so small we can't see it, and breast cancer? While mere speculation, what comes to my mind is, once again, bacteria.

Bacteria need three things to grow: heat (the right temperature range), moisture and food. Particle pollution, being made up of carbon, could be the perfect food that bacteria might use to grow and thrive. We breathe it in the air, it lodges in our lungs and from there, gets into the circulatory system, the blood. From there it can do its damage anywhere in the body. Why the link with the breasts per se? I do not know.

About a third of the explanation for the pattern of breast cancer deaths is due to air pollution, that dirt in the air from car and truck exhaust as well as from power plants that make our electricity. I was excited last night with the accomplishment of having "figured out" breast cancer, an exaggeration in my own mind, of course. But then, I was suddenly struck by fear for the girls and women whom I love, all exposed to higher than average levels of particle air pollution based on where they happen to be living.

In an attempt to keep that fear in perspective, I calmed myself by highlighting the following counter-points. First, particle pollution levels have come down according to an EPA (US government) analysis. For the 14 years between 2000 and 2013, levels of PM 2.5 (Particulate Matter 2.5 microns) (annual) have declined 34 percent. That is a decline of about 2.43 percent per year.

Over the past several decades since the start of the Clean Air Act in 1970, great strides have been made. Cars are becoming cleaner, less polluting, as the mileage per gallon increases, as best as I understand. By 2025, cars and light trucks might be able to get 54.5 miles per gallon which should result in even cleaner air.

Power plants are emitting less pollution as some in the Midwest have converted to natural gas as a result of the cost advantage since the price decline in oil and natural gas (subject to change over time, of course). This was the result of the industry revolution brought about by the inventions of fracking and horizontal drilling (Stephen Moore, lecture at Brown in about 2015).

While there is little information about air pollution historically, I believe it is safe to assume that, compared to the middle 1930s when my grandmother got breast cancer in the New York area, the air should be much cleaner. And yet, air pollution is still too high in many parts of the country. The point here is that it IS coming down, a great achievement over the decades which should eventually improve human health.

There is another reason to feel less frantic about this discovery about a strong link between particle air pollution and breast cancer. While cancer in general is, obviously, a major disease category, in the end, it only accounts for 23 percent of all deaths, under a quarter, during the years 2011-2013.

Furthermore, breast cancer is only a small portion of deaths from cancer during the period. It accounts for only 7 percent of all deaths from cancer in 2011-2013. To make it sound even less threatening, breast cancer, as a percent of ALL deaths, is only 1.6 percent - well under 2 percent - of all of the things from which people died in that set of years. Even given still high air pollution, the odds of any woman dying from breast cancer are still low.

Chapter 5. Colon Cancer and a Link with not Keeping One's Teeth Clean Enough

In 2014, about 50,310 people should have died from colorectal cancer based on an advanced estimate for that year. When I say "colon cancer", I am referring to the broader death category that includes cancer of the colon, rectum and anus. The annual death rate during the years 2011-2013 for the age 18 and over part of the population is 21.7 deaths per hundred thousand for the United States. Given that the cancer death rate is 241.4, "colon" cancer, as a percent of all cancer deaths, is 9 percent of the cancer total. As the death rate from all causes is 1047.0, colon cancer is 21.7/1047.0 or just about exactly 2 percent of all deaths in an average year during this three year period.

Table 5-1 is the colon cancer death rate by state (including of course, Washington DC, District of Columbia, called in the truncated 8 character state name list, District), the average annual rate during this period for this death category. It ranges from the lowest rate in Utah of about 13 deaths per hundred thousand people, to the highest rate in West Virginia of about 30 deaths. Compared to the highest death rate state, colon cancer death rates in the lowest state are 12.7/30.4 only 42 percent the size, or 58% less (100-42).

For colon cancer, I present three models with the final one being the one I consider best. I present all three because there is something we can learn from each. The decision about which is best combines technical considerations having to do with the method and theoretical matters about which model might teach us the most about colon cancer.

Before describing the first colon cancer model, I should note that older age (age 65 and over) appears in all three. Older age can be thought of as a "control", a somewhat arbitrary designation which suggests that our interest lies elsewhere. Older age is linked with dying from colon cancer, the most relevant cut off of those I checked (including age 85) being percent age 65 and over. The higher the percent of the population in a state in that age category, the more deaths from colon cancer.

The first colon model shows a link with not only older age but also obesity. We can become familiar with this new item in Table 5-2 - Obesity. Percent Obese in 2011. In a health survey, a person was asked their height and weight.

Table 5-1 Colon Cancer death rates
(colon, rectum, anus) by state 2011-2013.

State	Rate	State	Rate
Colorado	20.7	North Dakota	27.8
Hawaii	21.8	Georgia	28.0
Massachusetts	22.7	South Dakota	28.1
District	23.7	Maryland	28.3
New Jersey	23.7	Nebraska	28.4
California	23.8	Pennsylvania	28.6
Utah	24.4	Delaware	28.8
Connecticut	24.5	Iowa	29.0
New York	24.5	North Carolina	29.1
Nevada	24.5	Virginia	29.2
Montana	24.6	Tennessee	29.2
Arizona	24.7	Kansas	29.6
Wyoming	25.0	Ohio	29.6
Vermont	25.4	Missouri	30.3
Rhode Island	25.4	Texas	30.4
Minnesota	25.7	Kentucky	30.4
New Hampshire	26.2	South Carolina	30.8
New Mexico	26.3	Indiana	30.8
Washington	26.5	Arkansas	30.9
Florida	26.6	Oklahoma	31.1
Oregon	26.7	Michigan	31.3
Idaho	27.0	Alabama	32.0
Illinois	27.1	West Virginia	32.4
Alaska	27.4	Louisiana	33.4
Wisconsin	27.7	Mississippi	34.9
Maine	27.8		

This information was then plugged into an equation that calculates body mass index or BMI. The person would then be (anonymously) put into one of three categories based on how much fat is on their body, not measured, of course, but roughly estimated from the equation.

We can call these three categories low, medium and high. For this research, I used the "high" category called "obese". Coming up with accurate names for the three categories is a bit of a problem given that the lowest category, considered normal and healthy, cannot always be described thus with accuracy.

We can find the obesity item in Table 5-2, Percent Obese in 2011. These numbers for obesity by state are from the Center for Disease Control and Prevention, Behavioral Risk Factor Surveillance System 2011. It goes from a low in the state of Colorado of about 21 percent of the population in the obese category. The high is in the state of Mississippi where about 35 percent of the population is in the obese category that year (2011). According to the result in the first colon model (which we will shortly view), "obesity" is linked with colon cancer. The higher the percent obese in a state, the more deaths from colon cancer in that state.

In Table 5-3, we find the colon obesity model showing that connection. As usual we begin with the bottom box, Correlations, to see that the two items, age and obesity, are not related to each other, a good thing for the integrity of the model above. The bottom line, zero order correlations with colon cancer deaths themselves show both correlated with colon cancer. As obesity is the focus here, the correlation between obesity and colon cancer is .637**.

Moving next to the top box, we learn that the model explains 77.1 percent of the pattern between states in deaths from colon cancer, higher, actually, than the other two models (to be presented shortly). We move now to the middle box to see the statistic significance with these quite nice Sig values of .000 and t values used to calculate them, very large at about 8 for obesity (a minimum requirement being 2).

Next we move to the Beta column and see that the effect of age is stronger, explaining more of the pattern. If we wanted, we could next use the B column to construct a new colon cancer death rate list after holding age constant to look at the effect of obesity on cancer. Of course, we would do this by plugging in the mean value for older age as we let obesity vary state by state.

Table 5-2 - Obesity

Percent Obese in 2011

State	%	State	%
Colorado	20.7	North Dakota	27.8
Hawaii	21.8	Georgia	28.0
Massachusetts	22.7	South Dakota	28.1
District	23.7	Maryland	28.3
New Jersey	23.7	Nebraska	28.4
California	23.8	Pennsylvania	28.6
Utah	24.4	Delaware	28.8
Connecticut	24.5	Iowa	29.0
New York	24.5	North Carolina	29.1
Nevada	24.5	Virginia	29.2
Montana	24.6	Tennessee	29.2
Arizona	24.7	Kansas	29.6
Wyoming	25.0	Ohio	29.6
Vermont	25.4	Missouri	30.3
Rhode Island	25.4	Texas	30.4
Minnesota	25.7	Kentucky	30.4
New Hampshire	26.2	South Carolina	30.8
New Mexico	26.3	Indiana	30.8
Washington	26.5	Arkansas	30.9
Florida	26.6	Oklahoma	31.1
Oregon	26.7	Michigan	31.3
Idaho	27.0	Alabama	32.0
Illinois	27.1	West Virginia	32.4
Alaska	27.4	Louisiana	33.4
Wisconsin	27.7	Mississippi	34.9
Maine	27.8		

Table 5-3 One Colon Cancer Model: The Role of Obesity (more deaths).

Model Summary

Model	R	R Square	Adjusted R Square	Std. Error of the Estimate
1	.883[a]	.780	.771	1.5692

a. Predictors: (Constant), OBES2011, AGE65IN6

Coefficients[a]

Model		Unstandardized Coefficients		Standardized Coefficients	t	Sig.
		B	Std. Error	Beta		
1	(Constant)	-9.275	2.449		-3.787	.000
	AGE65IN6	1.216	.134	.619	9.050	.000
	OBES2011	.583	.074	.541	7.911	.000

a. Dependent Variable: COLON113

Correlations

		AGE65IN6	OBES2011	COLON113
AGE65IN6	Pearson Correlation	1	.154	.703**
	Sig. (2-tailed)	.	.279	.000
	N	51	51	51
OBES2011	Pearson Correlation	.154	1	.637**
	Sig. (2-tailed)	.279	.	.000
	N	51	51	51
COLON113	Pearson Correlation	.703**	.637**	1
	Sig. (2-tailed)	.000	.000	.
	N	51	51	51

**. Correlation is significant at the 0.01 level

I will not proceed with this given that this model was not chosen as the final and best one. Nevertheless, it is interesting to note that colon cancer is linked with obesity.

Why did the model fail to meet my test for being the best model? After all, it is the most successful one in terms of the amount of the pattern it explains (Adjusted R Square). Furthermore, the items are nicely uncorrelated, and the significance test shows the items solidly connected with colon cancer making us confident that the connection would hold in a larger population.

The problem with this obesity model is theoretical. While obesity is not quite a disease, it is, in many ways similar. This is so much the case that it appears to raise a question in my mind whether it is appropriate to use one "disease" as an explanation for another. Nevertheless, it is interesting to know that extra fatness on the body is linked with colon cancer, as if very overweight people needed more bad news about their situation.

Looking to other possible models now, in a second model, colon cancer is revealed to be linked with smoking. More smokers, more deaths from colon cancer. As this particular list for smoking is new in these models, I present the list in Table 5-4 Smokers. Percent Smokers in 1997. It goes from a low in the state of Utah of about 14 percent to a high in Kentucky of about 31 percent.

We can find the colon cancer - smoking model in Table 5-5. The bottom box shows no significant correlation between the items (no stars), a good thing. The bottom row shows clear zero order correlations with both items, the link between smokers and colon cancer being plus .556**, meaning more smokers, more deaths from colon cancer.

Moving to the top box now, the part of the pattern explained by this model is 67 percent (.670 Adjusted R Square). In the middle box, we see the significance of this simple two item model strongly and clearly. Sig. is recorded as .000 and t for smokers is over 5. If we wanted, we would use the actual equation summarizing the entire relationship found in the numbers in Table 5-1 Colon Cancer. We would control for age and see the effect of smoking on dying from colon cancer in the form of a new list of "predicted" numbers.

We learn from this second colon cancer model that here is another specific kind of cancer linked with smoking after lung cancer (in a model not shown). This corrects an impression from Chapter 2 that is not exactly right.

Table 5-4 Smokers
Percent Smokers in 1997

Utah	13.8		Vermont	23.3
California	18.4		South Carolina	23.4
Hawaii	18.7		Florida	23.6
District	18.8		Washington	23.8
Idaho	19.9		Wyoming	24.0
Maryland	20.4		Pennsylvania	24.2
Massachusetts	20.5		Rhode Island	24.3
Montana	20.5		South Dakota	24.3
Oregon	20.7		Virginia	24.4
Arizona	21.1		Louisiana	24.5
New Jersey	21.4		Oklahoma	24.6
Connecticut	21.6		New Hampshire	24.7
Minnesota	21.9		Alabama	24.7
New Mexico	22.1		Ohio	25.1
Nebraska	22.1		North Carolina	25.9
North Dakota	22.3		Michigan	26.0
Georgia	22.4		Indiana	26.4
Colorado	22.6		Alaska	26.5
Kansas	22.6		Delaware	26.6
Texas	22.6		Tennessee	26.9
Maine	22.7		West Virginia	27.4
New York	23.1		Nevada	28.1
Iowa	23.1		Arkansas	28.4
Mississippi	23.1		Missouri	28.6
Illinois	23.2		Kentucky	30.7
Wisconsin	23.2			

Table 5-5 A Second Colon Cancer Model:
The Role of Smoking (more deaths).

Model Summary

Model	R	R Square	Adjusted R Square	Std. Error of the Estimate
1	.826[a]	.683	.670	1.8864

a. Predictors: (Constant), SMOKRS97, AGE65IN6

Coefficients[a]

Model		Unstandardized Coefficients		Standardized Coefficients	t	Sig.
		B	Std. Error	Beta		
1	(Constant)	-4.702	2.694		-1.745	.087
	AGE65IN6	1.220	.162	.622	7.518	.000
	SMOKRS97	.489	.092	.442	5.340	.000

a. Dependent Variable: COLON113

Correlations

		AGE65IN6	SMOKRS97	COLON113
AGE65IN6	Pearson Correlation	1	.184	.703**
	Sig. (2-tailed)	.	.196	.000
	N	51	51	51
SMOKRS97	Pearson Correlation	.184	1	.556**
	Sig. (2-tailed)	.196	.	.000
	N	51	51	51
COLON113	Pearson Correlation	.703**	.556**	1
	Sig. (2-tailed)	.000	.000	.
	N	51	51	51

**. Correlation is significant at the 0.01 level (2-tailed).

In that chapter, when we removed lung cancer from all cancer deaths, smoking was no longer significantly linked with these other cancers. While still true when taken together, we now know that there is at least one additional cancer that IS connected with smoking – colon cancer. This is interesting although it is not exactly clear how smoking might be linked with more deaths from colon cancer. I will have more to say about that shortly.

It is now time to introduce an additional model for colon cancer which provides one more support column for what will eventually become the final model – a connection with not going to the dentist. The more people who say they went to the dentist over the past year, the FEWER the deaths from colon cancer.

"Dentist" can be found in Table 5-6. Percent who visited the dentist in the past year. The lowest percent is for West Virginia where about 53 percent say they went to the dentist. The highest is for Connecticut where about 79 percent say they were at the dentist over the past year.

The simple "dentist" model for colon cancer can be found in Table 5-7. It has two items. Older age, more deaths from colon cancer. As stated above a different way, more people going to the dentist over the past year, FEWER deaths from colon cancer.

Looking at the bottom Correlations box, no significant correlation between the items of older age and dentist. For zero order correlations, there is one between going to the dentist and colon cancer and the direction is negative (minus). More people who say they were at the dentist, fewer deaths from colon cancer.

These models show that both smoking and dentist are related to colon cancer. I was going to use the model for dentist in Table 5-7 as the final model. This is because it is so rich with new knowledge from a theoretical point of view. During the night, however, I reconsidered the matter deciding we needed one more model, a combination, showing both dentist and smoking.

The reason for this is that smoking and dentist happened to be somewhat linked with each other in a negative association. We can see this on the page for the final model now, Table 5-8: Colon Cancer Death Rates - The beneficial role of going to the dentist and the negative role of smoking.

Looking at the bottom Correlations box in Table 5-8, we see a negative association between smokers and dentist (-.440**). Yesterday, I thought we don't need the complication of such a correlation between items even though it is below the cutoff in size terms of .6. During the night, however, I realized the following problem.

Table 5-6 Dentist:
Percent who visited the dentist in the past year

State	%	State	%
West Virginia	53.1	Florida	68.8
Mississippi	57.1	Arizona	68.9
Oklahoma	57.8	California	69.0
Arkansas	58.5	Colorado	69.2
Louisiana	58.9	Oregon	70.2
Nevada	59.2	Pennsylvania	70.2
Alabama	60.1	Illinois	70.6
Kentucky	60.2	Iowa	70.8
Missouri	60.8	Alaska	71.1
Texas	61.7	Delaware	71.1
North Dakota	62.9	New York	71.2
New Mexico	64.2	District	71.4
Montana	64.3	Vermont	71.7
Georgia	64.7	Maryland	71.9
Wyoming	65.4	Nebraska	72.4
Idaho	65.7	Utah	72.9
Ohio	66.6	Minnesota	72.9
Indiana	66.6	New Hampshire	72.9
South Dakota	66.9	Virginia	73.1
Kansas	67.0	New Jersey	73.6
South Carolina	67.0	Rhode Island	75.4
North Carolina	67.1	Wisconsin	75.5
Maine	67.2	Massachusetts	75.9
Tennessee	67.5	Hawaii	77.0
Washington	67.9	Michigan	78.0
		Connecticut	79.1

Table 5-7 A Third Colon Cancer Model:
The Role of Not Visiting the Dentist (more deaths).

Model Summary

Model	R	R Square	Adjusted R Square	Std. Error of the Estimate
1	.838[a]	.703	.690	1.8265

a. Predictors: (Constant), DENTLVIS, AGE65IN6

Coefficients[a]

Model		Unstandardized Coefficients B	Std. Error	Standardized Coefficients Beta	t	Sig.
1	(Constant)	22.831	3.693		6.182	.000
	AGE65IN6	1.322	.155	.674	8.539	.000
	DENTLVIS	-.256	.044	-.457	-5.798	.000

a. Dependent Variable: COLON113

Correlations

		AGE65IN6	DENTLVIS	COLON113
AGE65IN6	Pearson Correlation	1	-.065	.703**
	Sig. (2-tailed)	.	.653	.000
	N	51	51	51
DENTLVIS	Pearson Correlation	-.065	1	-.501**
	Sig. (2-tailed)	.653	.	.000
	N	51	51	51
COLON113	Pearson Correlation	.703**	-.501**	1
	Sig. (2-tailed)	.000	.000	.
	N	51	51	51

**. Correlation is significant at the 0.01 level (2-tailed).

I am promoting this new finding that colon cancer is linked with not going to the dentist. How can we be certain, however, that this effect is not, to a large extent, due to smoking rather than to not going to the dentist if both are linked with each other? Given this connection, if I were to argue that going to the dentist was linked with colon cancer (in a negative direction), I had to be certain that this was not a misrepresentation due to the link between smoking and not going. The only way to do this was to have both in the model.

This final model for colon cancer appears in Table 5-8. It has three items, older age (as a control), going to the dentist, and smoking. Older age is linked with more deaths from colon cancer. Going to the dentist is linked with FEWER deaths. And smoking is linked with more deaths from colon cancer.

Reading the final Table 5-8, as we already noted, the correlation between dentist and smokers (negative in direction), we now glance at the final row, the zero order correlations between each item and colon cancer. For Smokers it is .556** and for dentist, it is -.501. Interestingly, in the final model above, the size order of these effects reverses (after accounting for age which is automatic from having it in the model).

Moving to the middle box now in Table 5-8, the two right columns show both items statistically significant with dentist at Sig. .000 with a t value of over 4.

Smokers, however, has a Sig .001 with a t value of 3.7. That is also an ok result but I note here that it is not perfect. This Sig. value of .001 might suggest a slight questioning of the solidness of the connection between smokers and colon cancer (after accounting this time for both age and dentist). This is relevant when we compare the solidness of this connection with the other items in terms of how certain we are that the connection from this so called sample applies to the larger population (of colon cancer at different times and in different places).

The Beta column shows the size order of each of the three items helping to account for the pattern of deaths across all the states. Older age is biggest, followed by the effect of dentist, and lastly, smoking.

We can roughly assess the size of the effects in relative terms from the Beta column in table 5-8. Adding the values together (without the decimals and ignoring the minus signs), we then divide each value by the total. Dentist, the effect of greatest interest, is thus 330/1252= 23.96 percent or about 24% of the part of the explanation that the model succeeds at illuminating.

Table 5-8 The Final Colon Cancer Model:
Not Going to the Dentist Plays a Role (more deaths)
Even After Accounting for the Role of Smoking (more deaths).

Model Summary

Model	R	R Square	Adjusted R Square	Std. Error of the Estimate
1	.878[a]	.771	.756	1.6207

a. Predictors: (Constant), SMOKRS97, AGE65IN6, DENTLVIS

Coefficients[a]

		Unstandardized Coefficients		Standardized Coefficients		
Model		B	Std. Error	Beta	t	Sig.
1	(Constant)	11.505	4.464		2.577	.013
	AGE65IN6	1.231	.139	.627	8.829	.000
	DENTLVIS	-.185	.044	-.330	-4.246	.000
	SMOKRS97	.327	.087	.295	3.737	.001

a. Dependent Variable: COLON113

Correlations

		AGE65IN6	DENTLVIS	SMOKRS97	COLON113
AGE65IN6	Pearson Correlation	1	-.065	.184	.703**
	Sig. (2-tailed)	.	.653	.196	.000
	N.	51	51	51	51
DENTLVIS	Pearson Correlation	-.065	1	-.440**	-.501**
	Sig. (2-tailed)	.653	.	.001	.000
	N.	51	51	51	.51
SMOKERS97	Pearson Correlation	.184	-.440**	1	.556**
	Sig. (2-tailed)	.196	.001	.	.000
	N.	51	51	51	.51
COLON113	Pearson Correlation	.703**	-.501**	.556**	1
	Sig. (2-tailed)	.000	.000	.000	.
	N.	51	.51	51	51

**. Correlation is significant at the 0.01 level (2-tailed).

We can also figure out the portion of the entire explanation that is explained by the model by taking into account that the total so far of 1252 is only 75.6 percent of the explanation (based on the Adjusted R Square). 1252/.756=x/1. 1252=.756x. X=1252/.756=1656.08. Now the value of the dentist Beta 330/1656.08=.199 or 19.9 percent of the total explanation for colon cancer. This means that almost 20 percent or a fifth of the total explanation of the colon cancer pattern across the states can be explained as from not going to the dentist.

As already noted briefly above, the total portion of the explanation for this pattern of colon cancer deaths is summarized in the top box of Table 5-8. The Adjusted R Square is .756 which means that the model as a whole accounts for 75.6 percent of the pattern.

Now we move to the actual equation created to represent the numbers for all the states in Table 5-1 Colon Cancer death rates.... This is found in the middle box in Table 5-8, the B column. We can use this now to come up with a more meaningful view of colon cancer deaths compared with the state death rates in Table 5-1.

Surely, we should hold constant older age, the least interesting, by using its mean value to accomplish this. Another easy decision is to "let vary" dentist, our most interesting result. We do this by telling the program to use the actual colon cancer death value for each state by putting into the equation the name of the item, in this case dentist, which I call [dentlvis] for dental visits.

The difficult decision here is what to do about smoking, whether to zero out its effect by using its mean, or whether to have it influence the death rate numbers by letting it vary. This decision is actually not that difficult. It is best to zero out the effect of smoking on death rates. Yes, very nice to know that smoking is linked with colon cancer, interesting mainly, as we already discussed, for the broader question of the role of smoking for getting cancer in general. We now know that smoking is linked with cancer not only because of lung cancer but also because of a link with colon cancer (so far).

Of course, we know from earlier (Chapter 2), this smoking effect for colon cancer is not strong enough for smoking to appear as a statistically significant effect for all the remaining kinds of cancer. Nevertheless, it still is interesting that it does appear as a solid and big enough effect to show up in the model for colon cancer by itself. As for why smoking might help lead to colon cancer, not that obvious, we will discuss shortly.

A second reason why smoking should be discounted in this "new look" is that it is a lifestyle factor and, so far, we have been more interested in the environment. For this model, however, it is not a good rationale because going to the dentist is not an environmental factor either and is also probably closer to a lifestyle item.

While still not an airtight distinction, in my own mind, I view smoking as an individual behavior that we either do or don't do which might not change based on where we lived. This is true even though Table 5-4 Smokers informs us that there is great variation between places in terms of how common it is for people to smoke (with a low of 14 percent smokers and a high of 32 percent). (This discussion ignores both the possible effect of second hand smoke, not in the model, as well as the quite plausible possibility that the percent of people smoking might influence how socially acceptable the habit is).

In the end, the decision to eliminate the effect of smoking (by zeroing it out in the equation) on the new look for colon cancer we are about to construct is due to the fact that we only needed it in the model to make clear that dentist was actually dentist and not smoking. The main interest, however, is dentist, the intriguing finding that not going is linked with dying from colon cancer.

Now with these decisions behind us, we can use the numbers in the B column in Table 5-8 to zero out the effect of two of the less interesting items, older age and smoking, while letting vary dentist, to get a nice view of its effect on the colon cancer death rate numbers.

To repeat how to do this, we zero out the two items by using their means in the equation and we let dentist vary by using the name of the dentist item [dentlvis]. We do this from the data box in SPSS 11, pulling down the window "Transform" and then highlighting "Compute". We will call this list coIndent, short for colon dentist. The equation follows below (using the numbers in the B column in Table 5-8). coIndent = 11.505 + (1.231 * 12.653) - (.185 * dentlvis) + (.327 * 23.396).

When running the equation, we get Table 5-9 CoIndent (Colon Dentist): The beneficial effect of going to the dentist on colon cancer death rates varying dentist (good) while holding constant older age (bad) and smoking (bad).

Table 5-9 Colndent (Colon Dentist):
The beneficial effect of going to the dentist on colon
cancer death rates varying dentist (good) while holding
constant older age (bad) and smoking (bad).

Connecticut	20.10	Washington	22.17
Michigan	20.30	Tennessee	22.24
Hawaii	20.49	Maine	22.30
Massachusetts	20.69	North Carolina	22.32
Wisconsin	20.76	Kansas	22.34
Rhode Island	20.78	South Carolina	22.34
New Jersey	21.12	South Dakota	22.35
Virginia	21.21	Ohio	22.41
Utah	21.24	Indiana	22.41
Minnesota	21.24	Idaho	22.58
New Hampshire	21.24	Wyoming	22.63
Nebraska	21.34	Georgia	22.76
Maryland	21.43	Montana	22.84
Vermont	21.47	New Mexico	22.85
District	21.52	North Dakota	23.09
New York	21.56	Texas	23.32
Alaska	21.58	Missouri	23.48
Delaware	21.58	Kentucky	23.59
Iowa	21.63	Alabama	23.61
Illinois	21.67	Nevada	23.78
Oregon	21.74	Louisiana	23.83
Pennsylvania	21.74	Arkansas	23.91
Colorado	21.93	Oklahoma	24.04
California	21.97	Mississippi	24.17
Arizona	21.98	West Virginia	24.91
Florida	22.00		

This view of colon cancer death rates for 2011-2013 is the most meaningful one with its focus on going to the dentist and its role in affecting death rates from colon cancer.

The predicted death rate is lowest in Connecticut at around 20 deaths, and highest in West Virginia at about 25 deaths. Compared to the highest death rate state, the death rate in the lowest state is only 81 percent the size. This means that, based on this one item, dentist, the death rate from colon cancer is lower by 19.3 percent or almost a fifth. This estimate of the size of the dentist effect on colon cancer death rates is rather close to the above estimate from the Beta column in Table 5-8 where we determined above that the size of dentist as a part of the total explanation is 19.9 percent or about a fifth.

How might we best interpret this finding that going to the dentist might reduce the death rate from colon cancer by about a fifth? The first thing that comes to mind is that it seems unlikely that it is going to the dentist itself that is responsible for this effect. Rather, it must be that the kinds of people who do not go are more likely to get cancer (for some reason).

To examine this alternative reasonable explanation, I checked education and income. Income is not a challenge of any kind but education is, rather unfortunately, a challenge to the dentist finding because it firstly, reduces the size of the significance to Sig. .005.

There is a zero order correlation between college and dentist of (minus) .518. The college item, not shown, is the percent of people in a state who have had any college. The higher that portion who have been to college, the higher the portion who have been to the dentist. Some of this dentist effect might, then, be due to the characteristics of people who attend college rather than due specifically to going to the dentist.

Again, unfortunately, college is linked as well to age, more people in the senior age group in a state, fewer people who have been to college (-.501), model not shown. In the end, while I note this information here, I chose not to include college in the final model due to these correlations which are a bit too high for me to feel comfortable. Furthermore, education is also linked with two other items.

I believe that the dentist finding is "real", that going to the dentist specifically, in some way, has an impact on whether or not people die from colon cancer. What could that be? The big problem is that people typically go to the dentist twice a year or even less often, among those who do go. In general, I like to stick as closely as possible to the simple meaning of the result.

For dentist, however, I think the best interpretation is a broader one which includes both the procedures the dentist performs in the office as well as posited encouragement which might promote oral hygiene activities at home.

Dentists clean the gums and teeth not to mention dealing with infections already present such as cavities (also called caries). The dentist mechanically gets under the gum-teeth interface to remove tartar and plaque. They also remove plaque from the surface of the teeth. Plaque is a biofilm composed of many kinds of bacteria. More and more recent articles keep increasing the number of strains of bacteria that live in the human mouth. First I read 100 kinds, then 200, and now 500.

What the dentist does during a visit might actually reduce the chances of dying from colon cancer with his or her mechanical disruption of bacteria on the teeth and in the area of the gums.

Because dental visits are so infrequent, there might also be an important role for "home care". We eat several times a day and it is the sugars from food that mix with saliva that are involved with causing the biofilm that needs to be mechanically removed (or chemically killed) on a regular basis. A visit to the dentist might encourage people to care for their teeth on a daily basis through education and encouragement. Any real effect on colon cancer of going to the dentist makes more sense when including greater adherence to teeth cleaning regimens at home.

How specifically might a "cleaner" mouth reduce the chances of dying from colon cancer? The broad result of the model suggests to me that "bad" bacteria from the mouth are involved in the development of colon cancer. As for the way these posited bad bacteria get from the mouth to the colon, it seems obvious that we swallow these microbes with food and drink and they end up in the digestive system making their way to and through the colon. A less direct possibility is that bad bacteria from the mouth may get breathed in and enter the bloodstream from the lungs. Once in the bloodstream, they can travel to many places in the body.

While this final point is beyond colon cancer, it is more well known that mouth bacteria play a role in heart disease. P. gingivalis, one strain involved with gum disease (gingivitis), has been found in the plaque removed from clogged arteries. This connection with another major disease makes a possible link with an important cancer more plausible.

In perhaps my only direct plug of the book, I believe that my commitment to using dental floss every day which started when I was age 49, might be the most important health activity I have ever done. At some point, I started doing it twice a day, including, of course, brushing with a manual toothbrush. A year or so ago, on the advice of my dentist (which I put into practice only after the passage of months), I discovered the Waterpik Water Flosser, Ultra model. I use that once a day to replace one time of manual flossing.

As a final topic, perhaps I should try and think how smoking might be linked with colon cancer. While not a direct focus of this study, it IS in the model and perhaps does deserve mention. It seems intuitively clearer for lung cancer how smoking might hurt the lungs. For colon cancer, it seems less obvious.

My tentative idea here is that smoking might lead to colon cancer by having a bad effect on the oral microbiota, the bacteria in the mouth. The matter is apparently difficult to pin down partly due to the "demographic" connection in the model itself between smokers and not going to the dentist. The negative correlation in this study and elsewhere suggests that smokers are themselves less likely to go to the dentist and through extension, probably less likely to engage in good oral hygiene activities at home.

It is difficult to untangle the "sociological" ways that smokers and non smokers might differ in terms of their backgrounds from any physical changes that smoking might cause in the mouth. There might be some direct physical effect of smoking on the mouth microflora that has an overall bad impact on general oral health. While this matter has been studied, there are conflicting results.

While it has not yet been shown definitively, I believe there is a good chance that smoking might make some dangerous bacterial strains in the mouth more likely to end up causing cancer in the colon. In sum, I believe that it is possible that smoking is linked with colon cancer by making the problem of bad mouth bacteria even more dangerous.

Chapter 6. Dying from Melanoma Linked with Having a Dog and with Not Strong Enough Ultraviolet

What I call here melanoma is a death category called Skin Cancer, with the technical name being Malignant melanoma of skin. The official name makes clear that it does not include other kinds of skin cancer that people die from although deaths from those cancers, basal and squamous cell carcinoma, are small. For this reason, the study here of melanoma has nothing to say about the causes of those other cancers of the skin (that usually do not lead to death).

The death rate from melanoma among the US population of all "races" during the years 2011-2013 for those age 18 and older was 3.9 deaths. All cancer deaths had a death rate of 241.4 and deaths from all causes, 1047.0. This means that melanoma deaths as a percent of all cancer deaths is 3.9/241.4= .016 or 1.6 percent. As a percent of all deaths during that period, the death rate from melanoma is 3.9/1047.0=.0037 or .37 percent of all deaths or a little more than a third of one percent. For these calculations, I use the period of 2011-2013 for comparison purposes with other cancers.

The model I end up presenting, however, is from the slightly earlier period of 2008-2010 for the technical reason that the melanoma value for Washington DC was missing due to their conclusion that the result was unreliable (probably because there were too few deaths). With only 51 cases in these models, we try to have a full set of numbers.

We start as usual with the Melanoma death rate by state in 2008-2010, Table 6-1. It ranges from a low of 1.4 deaths per hundred thousand people in "District", Washington DC, to a high of 5.3 deaths in West Virginia.

The final model has three items. The first is percent of households in a state that have one or more dogs. The more households with a dog, the more deaths from melanoma in that state. The second is our now familiar age item: seniors, the percent of people in the state who are age 65 or older. The more such people as a percent of the population in a state, the more deaths from melanoma. The third item is ultraviolet, one of three parts of sunlight including light (the part we can see), heat (called infrared) and ultraviolet, the part that can make our skin darker. The more ultraviolet that reaches the ground in the largest city of the state, the FEWER people die from melanoma in that state.

Table 6-1 melanoma.
Average yearly death rate from melanoma between 2008 and 2010 by state.

District	1.4	Utah	4.1
Hawaii	2.3	Washington	4.1
Alaska	2.7	Alabama	4.2
Georgia	3.0	Arizona	4.2
Texas	3.1	North Carolina	4.2
Mississippi	3.1	Montana	4.2
New York	3.1	Wyoming	4.3
Louisiana	3.2	Massachusetts	4.3
Illinois	3.3	Tennessee	4.4
California	3.4	Kansas	4.4
South Dakota	3.4	Missouri	4.5
North Dakota	3.4	Indiana	4.5
Nevada	3.5	Ohio	4.5
Minnesota	3.5	Colorado	4.6
Maryland	3.6	Oklahoma	4.6
Michigan	3.6	Kentucky	4.6
South Carolina	3.7	Pennsylvania	4.6
New Jersey	3.7	Iowa	4.6
Delaware	3.8	Florida	4.7
New Mexico	3.9	Idaho	4.8
Rhode Island	3.9	Nebraska	4.8
Connecticut	3.9	Maine	4.9
New Hampshire	3.9	Oregon	4.9
Arkansas	4.0	Vermont	5.1
Virginia	4.0	West Virginia	5.3
Wisconsin	4.0		

Now we can become familiar with these three lists which are a presentation of values for each state. Table 6-2 is dog, the percent of households with a dog (one or more). It ranges from a low in Washington DC (District) of about 7 percent of households to a high in Wyoming of about 48 percent of households with a dog.

Seniors can be found in Table 6-3, the percent age 65 and over in a state, familiar from earlier models. The lowest percent of seniors is in Alaska, about 7 percent (too cold?) and the highest is in Florida with about 17% of the population in the seniors category of age 65 or higher.

Lastly is ultraviolet in Table 6-4 which is the yearly average of the intensity of ultraviolet reaching the ground in the largest city of the state in 1996. In perhaps the greatest good fortune of the entire project, the UV Index government scientist most kindly agreed to construct for me a yearly average from the daily values for the UV Index for each of the big cities on the list.

This was in 1997 and his name, which I still remember, was Craig Long. Of course, I do not imply that he endorses the results of this project. (I, apparently, wrote this chapter before successfully contacting him a second time, almost twenty years later, when he constructed a new, nine year, average for ultraviolet intensity for later years in one large city for each state). This model uses the original list of ultraviolet for the year 1996, however.

The UV Index, based on satellite data, predicts for many large cities in the United States the intensity of ultraviolet in sunlight that will reach the ground the following day using such factors as cloud cover. While it is a prediction made less than a day in advance, I believe the estimate to be based on good science which includes a conversion of actual ultraviolet into a form that takes into account its effect on human skin before constructing the UV Index value. Thus, the science behind this daily value provides a good basis for a valid yearly measure for each city used in this analysis.

This UV index for a few decades now has been a part of the summer weather forecast on local TV and radio as it is often translated into how much time you can be at the beach before you get a sunburn. The number is in the range of 1 to 10 but it also goes higher in places with very strong sun. UV Index maps are available on the internet for the entire United States on a daily basis.

Table 6-2 dog.
Percent of households with a dog (one or more)

State	%	State	%
District	6.9	Alaska	34.0
New York	21.9	Washington	34.0
Massachusetts	22.5	South Dakota	34.3
Rhode Island	22.6	Arizona	34.4
New Jersey	23.1	Kansas	34.8
Connecticut	25.2	Nebraska	35.2
New Hampshire	25.5	Kentucky	35.4
Vermont	25.8	Louisiana	35.7
Maryland	26.6	Georgia	35.8
Maine	26.9	South Carolina	35.8
North Dakota	27.6	Alabama	35.9
Pennsylvania	27.7	Tennessee	36.0
Wisconsin	28.2	North Carolina	36.9
Florida	28.2	Missouri	36.9
Illinois	28.3	Mississippi	37.5
Minnesota	28.5	Nevada	37.8
Michigan	30.2	Colorado	38.1
Ohio	30.4	West Virginia	39.3
Delaware	31.2	Idaho	39.4
Virginia	31.3	Montana	40.0
Iowa	31.6	Texas	40.9
Utah	31.8	Arkansas	41.2
Hawaii	32.0	New Mexico	41.3
California	32.0	Oklahoma	41.7
Oregon	32.9	Wyoming	47.9
Indiana	33.6		

Table 6-3 Older Age.
Percent Age 65 and Over in each state (2006)

State	%	State	%
Alaska	6.8	New Jersey	12.9
Utah	8.8	Kansas	12.9
Georgia	9.8	Oregon	12.9
Texas	9.9	Wisconsin	13.0
Colorado	10.0	New York	13.1
California	10.8	Oklahoma	13.2
Nevada	11.1	Nebraska	13.3
Idaho	11.5	Massachusetts	13.3
Washington	11.5	Vermont	13.3
Virginia	11.6	Missouri	13.3
Maryland	11.6	Connecticut	13.4
Illinois	12.0	Delaware	13.4
Minnesota	12.1	Alabama	13.4
Wyoming	12.2	Ohio	13.4
North Carolina	12.2	Montana	13.8
Louisiana	12.2	Rhode Island	13.9
District	12.3	Arkansas	13.9
New Mexico	12.4	Hawaii	14.0
New Hampshire	12.4	South Dakota	14.2
Indiana	12.4	North Dakota	14.6
Mississippi	12.4	Iowa	14.6
Michigan	12.5	Maine	14.6
Tennessee	12.7	Pennsylvania	15.2
Arizona	12.8	West Virginia	15.3
South Carolina	12.8	Florida	16.8
Kentucky	12.8		

Table 6-4 [ultra96] ultraviolet in 1996.

UV Index (UVI) yearly average for the year 1996, the intensity of the ultraviolet in sunlight reaching the ground at solar noon in the largest city of the state.

Alaska	1.4	West Virginia	4.0
Washington	2.7	Idaho	4.0
Vermont	2.9	Kentucky	4.1
Oregon	3.0	Missouri	4.1
Maine	3.1	Virginia	4.4
North Dakota	3.1	North Carolina	4.6
New Hampshire	3.2	Utah	4.7
Minnesota	3.2	Kansas	4.7
Massachusetts	3.3	Wyoming	4.7
Wisconsin	3.3	Tennessee	4.8
Michigan	3.3	Arkansas	4.8
Rhode Island	3.4	Colorado	4.9
Connecticut	3.4	Georgia	5.1
Ohio	3.4	Oklahoma	5.2
Illinois	3.5	South Carolina	5.3
South Dakota	3.5	Mississippi	5.5
Montana	3.5	Nevada	5.7
New York	3.6	Alabama	5.8
Iowa	3.7	California	5.9
Indiana	3.7	Louisiana	5.9
Pennsylvania	3.8	Texas	5.9
Nebraska	3.8	New Mexico	6.1
New Jersey	3.9	Arizona	6.2
Maryland	3.9	Florida	6.9
Delaware	3.9	Hawaii	9.6
District	4.0		

We are ready to look now at Ultraviolet (the UV Index value averaged for the entire year of 1996) in Table 6-4. I use this available information of the UV Index for the
largest city in the state to represent the intensity of ultraviolet reaching the ground in the entire state. This is, of course, an imperfect, but apparently satisfactory, approximation for the state.

It ranges from the state with the lowest level of ultraviolet reaching the ground around noon time (solar noon) on a typical day which is Alaska with a UVI (UV Index) value of 1.4. This is perhaps not surprising looking at a map of the US and seeing just how far north Alaska really is compared to the rest of the "lower 48". Washington state is also very low with a UVI value of 2.7. This value is for Seattle, the largest city, very far north for the continental United States. On the east coast is Vermont, third lowest UV intensity with a UVI value of 2.9 over the course of the year.

Not surprisingly, Hawaii has the highest intensity of ultraviolet that reaches the ground on a typical day, a yearly UVI value of 9.6. Looking at the map makes us realize just how much farther south Hawaii is from the most southern state in the continental US, Florida, with a UVI value of 6.9. While this number is for the largest city, Miami, I stood at the buoy-shaped landmark in Key West, another some 5 hours drive south, which said "most southern place in the continental United States".

We are now ready to examine the final melanoma model in Table 6-5. As usual, we begin with the bottom box of correlations to make sure that, as much as possible, the items in the model are not correlated with each other or if they are, that the correlations are under the cutoff of .6. The items are uncorrelated with the exception of ultraviolet which is linked with dog +.326*. Apparently, there are somewhat more households with dogs as the sun becomes stronger (as we move south). While not ideal, this connection has a level of solidness of one star, thankfully not two, and the size is not too large.

While not essential, while we are in the lowest box, we glance at the bottom line to see that there is a zero order correlation between melanoma and two of the items, the bigger being with age (+.372**) (more seniors - more deaths from melanoma). There is a correlation between dying from melanoma and households with a dog as well, not so strong though (one star) (+.342*). More households with a dog, more deaths from melanoma.

For ultraviolet, there is no zero order correlation (with melanoma) meaning that whatever connection we find between the two only appears in the full model after we account for the effect of the other items.

Table 6-5 The Melanoma Model:

The Role of Having a Dog (more deaths)

and not strong enough ultraviolet (more deaths).

Model Summary

Model	R	R Square	Adjusted R Square	Std. Error of the Estimate
1	.690[a]	.476	.442	.5537

a. Predictors: (Constant), ULTRA96, AGE65IN6, DOGHOUSE

Coefficients[a]

Model		Unstandardized Coefficients		Standardized Coefficients	t	Sig.
		B	Std. Error	Beta		
1	(Constant)	.128	.770		.166	.869
	DOGHOUSE	6.253E-02	.012	.573	5.009	.000
	AGE65IN6	.225	.048	.509	4.687	.000
	ULTRA96	-.243	.063	-.437	-3.866	.000

a. Dependent Variable: MELA810

Correlations

		DOGHOUSE	AGE65IN6	ULTRA96	MELA810
DOGHOUSE	Pearson Correlation	1	-.175	.326*	.342*
	Sig. (2-tailed)	.	.220	.020	.014
	N	51	51	51	51
AGE65IN6	Pearson Correlation	-.175	1	.084	.372**
	Sig. (2-tailed)	.220	.	.560	.007
	N	51	51	51	51
ULTRA96	Pearson Correlation	.326*	.084	1	-.208
	Sig. (2-tailed)	.020	.560	.	.144
	N	51	51	51	51
MELA810	Pearson Correlation	.342*	.372**	-.208	1
	Sig. (2-tailed)	.014	.007	.144	.
	N	51	51	51	51

*. Correlation is significant at the 0.05 level (2-tailed).
**. Correlation is significant at the 0.01 level (2-tailed).

Given the correlation of ultraviolet and dog, this is the one that must likely be taken into consideration before the link between ultraviolet and melanoma becomes apparent.

Further extending the same point, we will learn in a moment that having a dog has a big impact on the overall model. Therefore, it makes sense that we might see the role of ultraviolet only after first taking the dog result into account.

While not a perfect result from the standpoint of validity, it is in the reasonably acceptable range and also makes sense from the perspective of the benefits of doing a model with more than one explanation, a multivariate model. We can see the influence of some items only after taking into account the influence of other items first.

Now we can move to the top box in Table 6.5 to check the total explanatory power of the model as a whole, the Adjusted R Square. It is .442 which means that the model accounts for 44.2% of the total explanation, the pattern of variation in the death rate numbers across all of the states. In the context of my typical models, this is very low. I selected this particular model from among many possibilities nevertheless because of its acceptable technical attributes combined with its interesting insights into melanoma that could represent new information. I would place this in the category of theoretical considerations.

In the middle box of Table 6-5, we have the main model for deaths from melanoma. As usual, we start with the statistical test in the two right columns to assess the solidness of the results. The Sig. values are .000, very solid, and the t values used to calculate the Sig. are well above 2, dog being over 5, and ultraviolet being 3.8.

Next is the size of each effect which we find in the Beta column of this middle box in the same Table 6-5. Dog is the biggest effect of the model and it is noteworthy that the effect of households with a dog is larger than that of older age. Ultraviolet is the smallest effect of the three but, as we will see in a moment, not really that small.

To further assess the size of these items on deaths from melanoma, we add the numbers in the Beta column together (ignoring negative signs and decimals): 573+509+437=1519. Of the part of the explanation for which the model accounts, dog explains 573/1519=.377, about 38 percent of the pattern. Age 65 explains 509/1519=.335 or about 34 percent of the pattern. Ultraviolet explains 437/1519=.288 or about 29 percent of the pattern.

As the model as a whole only explains about 44 percent of the total pattern, we want to reduce the size of these numbers to learn what portion of the TOTAL pattern imbedded in these death rate numbers is explained by each of the items. 1519/.442=x/1. 1519=.442x. x=1519/.442. x=3436.65. That is the new denominator and now, each beta value can be divided by that number.

For dog: 573/3436.65=.167. Households with dogs explains some 17 percent of the total pattern. Percent seniors explains 509/3439.65=.148 or around 15 percent of the total pattern of difference between states in deaths from melanoma. Lastly, ultraviolet explains 437/3436.65=.127, or about 13 percent of the total pattern of deaths from melanoma across all the states.

Lastly is the equation itself, a numerical representation of the pattern of melanoma deaths across the states. This can be found in the B column of the middle box in Table 6-5. We will use this now to come up with a new look of the pattern of melanoma deaths by "zeroing out" the items in which we are less interested so we can focus on the items of interest. As you might now recall, we can do this by replacing the actual value for each state of the item of less interest with its average value (mean). We can use the actual state value only for the items of interest.

What might this most interesting view of melanoma look like? For me, it seems obvious. While it is quite interesting finding a connection with having a dog, something we will discuss in a moment, either a person lives in a household with a dog or does not. The link between older age and deaths from melanoma is not surprising even though it surely has to be in the model as a control. Repeating from past chapters, death is more likely to be visited upon the older among us and this is particularly the case with dying from cancer.

Clearly, the most interesting to me is ultraviolet, the finding that the less strong the ultraviolet that reaches the ground at mid day during a typical day, the more people die from melanoma. For this selected view, then, we can zero out the effect of dog and of older age in order to see more clearly the effect of ultraviolet. This will give us a "predicted" death rate for melanoma by state for this set of years.

This best view would only represent a small portion of the total explanation. We learned above that the size of this portion is about 13 percent. Further, the ordering of states in this new list would be identical to the ordering of states in Table 6-4 Ultraviolet (because this is the only item that we are allowing to vary). Nevertheless, it is worth constructing this new list in order to see from the perspective of actual numbers how the death rate from melanoma is affected by this item of interest, variations from state to state in the intensity of ultraviolet that reaches the ground in sunlight.

After this explanation, we are now ready to set up the equation from the B column, middle box in Table 6-5. While the equation works fine with the B value as written for age, I will change it to a form more familiar, from 6.253E-02 to .06253. We write the equation in SPSS 11 from the data file pulling down "transform" and highlighting "compute". We add in the means for the two less interesting items: dog mean 32.406 (average percent of households with a dog across all the states is about 32 percent) and older age mean: 12.643 (average percent seniors is about 13 percent). For the item of interest, ultraviolet, we put in the name of the item "ultra96" which tells the program to use the actual number for ultraviolet for each state.

The equation for this best view is as follows. We will call it (with the 8 character maximum): melasun. melasun = .128 + (.06253 * 32.406) + (.225 * 12.643) - (.243 * ultra96).

This "best view" melanoma list of state death rates can now be found in Table 6-6 Melasun. Predicted death rates from melanoma by state showing the beneficial effect of ultraviolet holding constant households with dogs (more, bad) and older age (bad) while letting vary ultraviolet (good). This best view list in Table 6-6 is the exact reverse of the ultraviolet list in Table 6-4 because more ultraviolet is linked with fewer deaths from melanoma in the model.

In the best view look of Table 6-6 melasun, Hawaii is the state with the lowest death rate, matching the fact that Hawaii is the bottom state on the ultraviolet list (Table 6-4), the state with the strongest ultraviolet. Conversely, Alaska is the state with the highest predicted melanoma death rate (with Washington state second highest), exactly matching in reverse the weaker intensity of ultraviolet reaching the ground in Table 6-4 for both of these states.

In Table 6-6, the predicted death rate from melanoma (due to the effect of ultraviolet) goes from a low of 2.67 deaths in Hawaii to a high of 4.66 in Alaska. Compared with this death rate in Hawaii, in Alaska, it is higher by about 75 percent. (2.67/100=4.66/x. 2.67x=466.

Table 6-6 melasun. Predicted death rate from melanoma after setting aside the effects of having a dog (more deaths) and older age (more deaths) in order to see the possible effect of insufficiently strong ultraviolet in sunlight on death rates (more deaths).

Hawaii	2.67	New Jersey	4.05
Florida	3.32	Maryland	4.05
Arizona	3.49	Delaware	4.05
New Mexico	3.52	Pennsylvania	4.08
California	3.57	Nebraska	4.08
Louisiana	3.57	Iowa	4.10
Texas	3.57	Indiana	4.10
Alabama	3.59	New York	4.12
Nevada	3.61	Illinois	4.15
Mississippi	3.66	South Dakota	4.15
South Carolina	3.71	Montana	4.15
Oklahoma	3.74	Rhode Island	4.17
Georgia	3.76	Connecticut	4.17
Colorado	3.81	Ohio	4.17
Tennessee	3.83	Massachusetts	4.20
Arkansas	3.83	Wisconsin	4.20
Utah	3.86	Michigan	4.20
Kansas	3.86	New Hampshire	4.22
Wyoming	3.86	Minnesota	4.22
North Carolina	3.88	Maine	4.25
Virginia	3.93	North Dakota	4.25
Kentucky	4.00	Oregon	4.27
Missouri	4.00	Vermont	4.29
District	4.03	Washington	4.34
West Virginia	4.03	Alaska	4.66
Idaho	4.03		

x=466/2.67. x=174.53). Done the other way, compared with the high death rate in Alaska, the death rate in the lowest state of Hawaii is only 57 percent as large. This means that the death rate in Hawaii from melanoma is 43 percent smaller than in Alaska.

I am surprised that the size difference in the predicted melanoma death rate is as large as it is given the small absolute size of ultraviolet as a portion of the total explanation. I checked the calculations, however, and they appear to be correct.

With the numbers portion of this melanoma analysis behind us, it is now time to try and comment on these surprising results. Looking at the model in Table 6-5, there is little more to be said about the link with older age, the middle item.

The first item, dog, comes as a surprise. To repeat the basic observation from earlier chapters, this study does not compare households with and without dogs so that we may be a little more certain about how to interpret the result here. These are all characteristics of states. States with more people living with dogs have more deaths from melanoma. (The more exact finding is that the more households there are that include one or more dogs, the more deaths there are from melanoma in that state per hundred thousand people). As with such results earlier, we assume here that this is because it is the people living with dogs who are more likely to die from melanoma (but we cannot be absolutely sure, perhaps stating the case too strongly). Assuming this to be true, the next question is why.

How would it be that people who live with a dog get melanoma and die from it? I never had a dog so my level of general knowledge is probably lower than average. I know from talking with other people that, unfortunately, dogs do get cancer and often die of it. How that might translate to humans getting cancer, I do not know.

Again with this disconcerting connection, I apologize to the many people who deeply love their pets repeating that it saddens me to have found this connection between dogs and melanoma.

Other models not shown here have suggested a link between melanoma and cats, households with one or more cats. Overall, I believe the link with dogs to be stronger but the matter is confusing because there is a correlation between dogs and cats. States with a higher percent of households who have a dog also have a higher percent of households with a cat. It is unclear whether these are the same or different households.

Lastly is the intriguing and controversial finding about ultraviolet. The model shows a link between the two but in a direction opposite to what one might expect. In light of its controversial nature, a number of careful caveats are perhaps in order.

First is the repetition about the scope of this research including only deaths from melanoma. This has nothing to say about the more common forms of skin cancer from which people do not typically die.

Second, the focus here is on deaths rather than incidence (getting it) and most people with melanoma never die from it. Might it be possible that what causes melanoma is different than what kills people from it? While this is unlikely, I do raise the possibility that having it and dying from it might not have the same "determinants". I admit, however, that this distinction is weak because you first have to have it in order to die from it and it is likely that the determinants are overlapping in each case.

Third, while I figure it was a matter of very good fortune to obtain the information necessary for these numbers on ultraviolet reaching the ground over the course of the entire year converted to a typical day of the year, this is ultimately a "macro" measure. No attempt is made here to measure actual exposure to the ultraviolet of the sun, a different kind of project that is more "micro" in nature. I assume that people typically get what they call "incidental exposure" to sunshine and its ultraviolet when walking from the store to the car, etc.

There is great variation in people's patterns of sun exposure, however. As one example, I was shocked to visit elderly friends in south Florida with its strong sunshine seeing that they were both "as white as ghosts". Despite these many unknowns, the stronger point is that people living at more northern latitudes where the ultraviolet barely reaches the ground over the course of the year (like Alaska) never have a chance for their bodies to be exposed in the first place. Despite this drawback of not measuring actual exposure, I do believe that this macro-level measurement of ultraviolet that reaches the ground is an indicator of ultraviolet hitting the human body in different geographic locations, particularly on an aggregate level of large groups of people.

Fourth is the possible difference between the ultraviolet portion of the sun and the two other parts (light and infrared). Perhaps we are jumping to conclusions (not yet discussed) that, by finding ultraviolet linked with fewer deaths from melanoma - that sun might actually good for you.

There is a mix of all three parts of sunlight that does not stay exactly the same. While the portion of ultraviolet in sunlight is about five percent, it varies, probably based on the strength of the ultraviolet portion from perhaps a low of three percent to a high of seven percent. This is mainly affected by latitude with the stronger-sun-places having a higher portion of ultraviolet. As far as sunlight reaching the ground, the only relevant matter for here is that variation is further affected by different filters of ultraviolet such as clouds. Other filters of ultraviolet include air pollution, such as ozone, well known to filter ultraviolet, but also particle pollution (based on my own observations using a UV meter and knowing the real-time level of particulate matter 2.5 microns).

Furthermore, in terms of human exposure, glass as in a car's side door, causes a further differential filtering of sunlight reducing the level of ultraviolet in the mix. I believe that all of these kinds of filters add to the variation in the starting sunlight mix based on the particular latitude. These filters differentially reduce ultraviolet and subsequently, increase the role of the infrared portion in sunlight.

The simple explanation of the finding here is that lower ultraviolet leads to more melanoma deaths because the strength of the general sunlight is also lower. There is room for a contrary interpretation, however, due to the possibility that the mix in sunlight is changed once ultraviolet is reduced in strength. If reduced ultraviolet strength is linked with melanoma cancer deaths, maybe this is because of the changed nature of sunlight which is now more purely infrared. Perhaps it is this altered infrared portion which increases deaths from melanoma.

I have been in Seattle Washington in summer and that sun, despite its relatively low ultraviolet, has an unusually burning feel to it. So perhaps it is sunlight depleted, for whatever reason, of a portion of its ultraviolet which might be the damaging factor that leads to melanoma in more northern places as well as in places with bad air pollution.

I have actually considered this to be a real possibility for many, many years, avoiding the late afternoon sun because the ultraviolet peaks early, near "solar" noon leaving the heat to dominate in the sun of the late afternoon. So perhaps, it is this "hot" sunshine from various causes that makes melanoma, a possibility that fits fine with the result here that weaker ultraviolet is linked with more melanoma deaths.

While I am far from ready to abandon this idea that ultraviolet-depleted sunshine might be dangerous, I fear it does not stand up as a good explanation for the findings here about melanoma.

It is at least worth trying to test the idea empirically as best as we are able. There are two problems to start with. One idea is to find ways to represent other parts of the sun now that we have ultraviolet. The problem is that the various parts of the sun are highly correlated with each other making it difficult (but not impossible) to test them in the model. For this reason we have to test various ideas of the ultraviolet-depleted sunshine hypothesis twice, one by itself putting it in the model without ultraviolet due to the proscription against having highly correlated items together in the same model. Then, we can test them a second time with ultraviolet as well. A simple test of finding the percent of ultraviolet in sunlight over the course of the year for each big city is a hopeless goal.

As I stated earlier, ultraviolet is the smallest portion of sunlight, around 3-7 percent, (my own estimate), and we have a set of numbers for that. Visible light is 40 plus percent. Even though energy from ultraviolet is much stronger, energy from the heat part of the sun or infrared is the largest part. We cannot see infrared but we can feel it indirectly when we walk by a brick building in summer that has been heated by the sun. We can now test these other parts of sunlight (as best as we are able) in the melanoma model.

One imperfect test for the infrared portion is total sun energy is called solar insolation. There are apparently these sun collectors all over the country that record this over the course of the year and I have a list of numbers for the yearly output of sun energy. Given that infrared represents a majority of this total sun energy, insolation is not bad as a test for the infrared portion. While I report these supplementary tests here, I will not present the results in detail.

As would be expected, the correlation between ultraviolet [ultra96] and sun insolation [suninsol] is a high .897. They cannot, therefore be tested at the same time in the model. Replacing ultraviolet with total sun energy, solar insolation, [suninsol] is not significant at the .01 level (Sig. .079). While in the original model, ultraviolet IS related to melanoma, total sun energy is NOT.

A second test is air temperature, an indirect way to measure the effect of infrared radiation. The sun's heat energy indirectly heats up the air. The temperature measure is the average temperature over the course of the entire day across the year, for 30 complete years, this one being for the period 1961-1990 (in the largest city of the state). It is called [temeanlv], which stands for temperature mean las vegas (as this older measure used Reno which I replaced given the tremendous growth of Las Vegas). Its correlation with ultraviolet is +.872**. Replacing ultraviolet with air temperature, seen here as connected with the infrared portion of the sunlight, shows an intriguing significant result Sig .005. Temperature seems as well to be connected with melanoma deaths. Hotter temperature, FEWER melanoma deaths.

This result bodes poorly for the ultraviolet-depleted sunlight hypothesis suggesting that the infrared in sunlight is causing melanoma. This is because the result here suggests the opposite. The higher the air temperature (heated indirectly by sunlight), the fewer the deaths from melanoma. (We would expect more deaths with more heat).

Now for a "battle of the Titans" between ultraviolet and infrared (air temperature). Which is it really as they are so closely linked with each other? Having them both in the model gives a clear answer. Temperature drops out (Sig. .586). Ultraviolet is clearly stronger. Overall, the result conflicts with the idea that it is really infrared behind the connection we are seeing in the model.

Lastly is visible light represented in lumens by the average yearly value for visible light in the largest city of the state called in my data [light]. It is correlated with ultraviolet +.872**, not at all surprising. Adding it to the model now first without ultraviolet, it is not significantly related to melanoma, Sig. .014, above the .01 threshold. With ultraviolet back in, light now clearly drops out - Sig. .313.

As far as melanoma is concerned, after the tests with the three components of sunlight including ultraviolet, however imperfect the test for infrared, we can conclude now with somewhat greater confidence. The connection for melanoma is with ultraviolet specifically. Given the high correlation between all three parts of sunlight, the near misses of the other parts are not surprising, all in the same negative direction. Overall, however, the result makes us more confident that the clearest and strongest connection for melanoma is with the ultraviolet component of sunlight.

Perhaps even more striking is the result with air temperature showing an alternative model connecting air temperature with melanoma. It is in the wrong direction, however, as we were thinking of explaining the original model result as really a connection with heat, infrared. It turns out, however, that infrared is unlikely to be a determinant of melanoma (more of it, more deaths) because the connection is in the other direction. When there is less warm air, there is a higher death rate from melanoma.

In my opinion, this is rather strong evidence that the heat explanation for the main finding is NOT correct. It seems that we are left with the simple explanation for this finding. It is ultraviolet specifically that is connected with melanoma and that this connection is in a negative direction. (In Table 6-5, Beta column, there is a minus sign in front of the ultraviolet result). The LOWER the ultraviolet, the higher the death rate from melanoma. Good God!

There is another conundrum worth mentioning. There is an idea that ultraviolet is responsible for melanoma because of sunburns in childhood. Clearly, the research here is not well suited for checking this possibility. As the case for all the models, deaths are recorded in the state where they occur and there is a huge amount of moving between states that occurs over the life cycle in the United States (also called internal migration).

While some move for work opportunities, a huge number move at the time of retirement, typically from the colder to the warmer and sunnier states. I was never aware of how widespread this pattern was until a friend, who did his dissertation on the topic, informed me that such was the case. While part of this involves being freed from the constraints of working, I personally suspect that health insurance has a great deal to do with this. Medicare, the health insurance program for seniors, is national in scope. I also believe that moving to a lower state-income-tax state, including many states with zero state income tax, is a factor. An additional tax matter is the extra state inheritance taxes (at the time of death) which are absent in many of the magnet states.

If the real cause of melanoma is events that occurred in childhood (at the local beach) and then the same person moves to another state and dies there, it is almost impossible to map this in the context of this research. That person is only included in the death rate where the person might have moved (as a senior) and died.

While this situation can apply to many diseases, I believe the general success of these statistical models diminishes the possibility that such is the case. Rather, it is more likely that dying from any particular disease is from events that occurred in the state of death itself. In the case of the many seniors who move upon retirement, this means their new adopted state such as Florida, Arizona or Nevada. In this case, were dying from melanoma truly from events during childhood (sunburns at that time), there would be little way these models could work.

I wish I could say more about the large-in-size finding linking dogs and melanoma. While surely disturbing to the 32 percent of households living with a dog, the best I can say is to emphasize that dying from melanoma is a quite rare occurrence, well under one percent of all deaths in a given year.

I have something else to say about the meaning of the ultraviolet finding. I was expecting to have a result showing a null finding between ultraviolet and melanoma, no connection. Were this the case, I was ready to conclude in the language of science that there was no evidence in this study to support the conclusion that melanoma was linked with ultraviolet.

The stronger result here leaves no choice but to make the concluding words stronger than that. There is a connection between ultraviolet and melanoma but it turns out to be in the OPPOSITE direction of what we thought. The more ultraviolet that reaches the ground, the FEWER the deaths from melanoma. Given this result, we can conservatively conclude that it is unlikely that ultraviolet is responsible for a higher death rate from melanoma.

Two days ago, I met a couple at Starbucks here to drop off their daughter for a university summer program. They were Swedish, about 50 or so, and have lived in Seattle Washington for the past 30 years. I happened to mention that I was working on melanoma and the woman lifted the bottom of her cuff to reveal a melanoma patch on her calf telling me that she had it. It shocked me as it was the first time I ever saw it in person. I could never be a cancer doctor and my hat is off to those who deal with these diseases up close on a daily basis.

I felt quite bad about it and it motivated me to redouble my efforts to come up with the best result that I was able to in the hope of bringing the day a little closer when we might defeat such diseases. It also reminded me not to play it safe as I was ready to do by selecting a different model because we are talking about people's lives. I dedicate this chapter to that lovely woman from Seattle and hope she will be all right.

While I thought that was it, during the night, I realized there was something important to add. It is about the specific nature of the ultraviolet item. I have known for many years that, if there would ever be success with this UV Index measure, it would be because of my rare good fortune that the kind government researcher was able to construct for me upon request, a YEARLY AVERAGE of daily UV Index scores for each location.

I realized in the past day that there is another reason for the degree to which the model is successful (showing a link between insufficiently intense ultraviolet and more deaths from melanoma). It has to do with the unusual nature of the ultraviolet measure based as it is on the daily prediction of ultraviolet reaching the ground in each location.

The many steps involved in calculating this daily prediction of ultraviolet are briefly summarized in an internet EPA sheet called "Calculating the UV Index". The UV Index in the United states is calculated by the U.S. National Weather Service. There is a daily map with UV Index numbers for different locations across the country (including Alaska and Hawaii and even Puerto Rico) as well as a companion list of UV Index values for large cities.

Returning to the way the UV Index is calculated, there is one detail that stands out in particular. As the purpose of the measure is to reflect the biological effect of ultraviolet on human beings, specifically its effect on human skin, different portions of the UV spectrum are "weighted", given a greater emphasis in the calculation to reflect the fact that they contribute more strongly to the reddening of human skin called "sunburn" or "skin damage" in the EPA description.

As I understand it, such reddening initiates a biological process which takes about 2 days to complete both in the skin and inside the body involving damage and repair, the speeding up of the cell cycle as well as the production of the hormone Vitamin D in the blood.

This weighted result is still a representation of ultraviolet reaching the ground and it does include the full ultraviolet spectrum from 280 to 400 nm (nanometers). This is often divided up into UVB (280-314 nm) and UVA (315-400 nm), this from the EPA sheet describing the way the UV index is calculated.

Nevertheless, it is not a direct measure of ultraviolet reaching the ground in a location but rather a measure of this once it has been transformed by giving different weights to varying parts of the spectrum based on the role each plays in creating a biological reaction in human skin called "sunburn".

It is my strong hunch that whatever success that the model here demonstrates linking ultraviolet to death from melanoma in a direction different than expected is largely due to this unusual transformation which shifts the focus to the biological effect on human skin. As an aside, there is a similar kind of measure geared to biological effect in the field of exposure to ionizing radiation.

Might the nature of this transformed measure that is the UV Index provide an opening for another contrarian interpretation of the main result in the model? After all, the focus on sunburn in human skin gives a larger weight to UV wavelengths in the stronger B range while reducing the influence of wavelengths in the weaker A range. In the random example of weights on the EPA sheet, (which are not actual weights), the 290nm wavelength (solidly in the strong B range) is given a weight of 15 while the 400nm wavelength (in the weakest part of the A range) is given a weight of 3. Perhaps this UV Index measure, by its weighting for its ability to cause reddening of the skin, gives an overemphasis to the B portion of the spectrum and an underemphasis to the A portion.

As this is likely true, might it not be possible that a lower UV index score is reflecting both diminished UVB as well as increased UVA as a portion of total ultraviolet due to the lesser ability of UVA to cause reddening in human skin? If so, then perhaps deaths from melanoma are increased when the yearly UV index score is low in a location because of exposure to sunlight in northern areas with this ultraviolet that is overly in the UVA range. Put more simply, could not the model result suggest that UVA is causing an increase in deaths from melanoma (as has surely been suggested before)?

The logic of this argument has its similarity to the previous challenge of ultraviolet-diminished sunlight. This time, the idea is sunlight whose UVA portion has been enhanced by the weakness in its B portion in more northern areas (of the northern hemisphere).

This challenging interpretation needs to be addressed. While the matter is, admittedly, a bit confusing, this challenge, like the previous one, probably does not stand up to scrutiny being too nuanced and small in size to be a reasonable explanation of the model result. While, of course, every reader is entitled to one's own opinion on the question, I will present my own thinking.

Changes in the proportion of the B and A parts of ultraviolet would have a relatively minor impact for the simple reason that, generally speaking, parts of sunlight are highly correlated with each other. As we drive from Florida to Maine, from San Diego California to Seattle Washington, all portions of sunlight get weaker together when seen from the view of the entire year. The heat part of the sun gets weaker, infrared, and the average temperature of the air gets colder. The light part of sunlight also apparently gets weaker during the entire year as we move away from the equator, toward the north. My [light] measure in lumens is correlated with latitude (minus) -.757**. Latitude numbers go higher as we look north on the map while total yearly light in a city gets dimmer (hence the negative correlation).

As for ultraviolet, the yearly UV Index measure in this study gets weaker and weaker as we move from south to north, obvious from a glance at the numbers in Table 6-4. As for the portions of ultraviolet reflected in the UV Index, the focus on this alternative possibility for interpreting the model result, this part is a bit speculative. Most would probably agree that a smaller yearly UV index number would mean that UVB is diminished as it is probably the main driver of the Index score.

How about UVA? While it is not possible to know for sure, it is very likely that the yearly total of UVA is also diminished in size. This would be true even if it increased as a portion of total ultraviolet. If absolute levels of UVA were diminished as the UV Index score dropped in size, even if it increased as a portion of total UV, we would be hard pressed to explain the model result after surmising this circumstance from the high correlation between the intensity of different portions of sunlight. If the intensity of UVA were weaker as is likely the case with a lower yearly UV Index score, it would be difficult to posit a role for weakened UVA as a determinant of melanoma deaths.

In this discussion of the role of UVA specifically, the research here is, in the final analysis, not designed to definitely address this matter. This is because the UV index includes the entire ultraviolet spectrum and does not estimate separate effects for each section of the UV spectrum grouped in the two categories that are reflected in the final predicted estimate of the index value at the high point of the day (around noon).

While I dislike broaching the subject of "indoor tanning", might this have any implications for the role of indoor tanning in deaths from melanoma? Electric tanning machines using bulbs that gave off radiation that caused the skin to redden was, I believe, invented in the United States in the 1930s or 1940s. I once saw a picture of Russian school children standing around an ultraviolet lamp during winter. We even had a basic tanning lamp at home growing up in the 1960s, a simple bulb with an aluminum reflector that clipped on to a table edge and plugged in, of course. We had to be careful because it was easy to burn. At some point later, perhaps in the 1970s, the concern arose that tanning wrinkled the skin and worse, might cause cancer.

Around this time perhaps, this concern found its way into government regulation of tanning machines in Europe as well as in Canada. (The United States was a slightly later arrival to the regulatory impulse). Likely due to these regulations, whose purpose was protecting public safety and health, tanning bulb manufacturers reduced the "stronger" sunburn-inducing parts of the ultraviolet spectrum in the B range to well below that of the natural sun leaving the A part which apparently worked to confer some skin color at high enough intensity.

That is the situation as it stands today with many recent tanning machines having a UVB portion of around 2 percent, lower than the typical outdoor sun which is around 5 percent. Due to the belief that indoor tanning is dangerous for health, there is now a US federal tax on tanning visits as part of the President Obama-era health care legislation. The Republican Congress had considered eliminating this as part of its "repeal and replace" revision but this has not occurred as of late October, 2017.

Is indoor tanning safe or might it be implicated in the development of melanoma years later and possible death from the same? My thoughts on this matter would be of limited utility because I have never attempted to see if I might be able to develop a macro test of the pattern of indoor tanning across the United States and to test it in the model here for melanoma deaths. Nevertheless, I have decided to raise the subject as a way to further develop the implications of the model result here.

If indoor tanning, especially popular among girls during their teen years, would lead to melanoma and death but only several decades later, this connection would be inherently difficult to uncover in a model like this. There is too much mobility in American society as so many have already moved states by their older years making such a link on a state level difficult to examine.

This research result on a state level, that lower yearly levels of ultraviolet are linked with more deaths from melanoma, implies that the connection between indoor tanning and melanoma is unlikely. There are two reasons why such is the case.

Firstly, as in the case above with overly rich portions of ultraviolet UVA in natural sunlight at northern latitudes, the same applies for artificial tanning machines. The altered spectrum of many indoor tanning machines, increasing the A portion within the range of ultraviolet, seems to be unnatural and I am not surprised others would tag it as dangerous. In the context of this research result on melanoma, however, this seems unlikely because melanoma deaths increase the lower the ultraviolet, not the higher. While this overemphasis on the A part of the spectrum is a somewhat different situation, since portions of the sunlight are correlated with each other, a higher level of one portion, the A part of ultraviolet would be unlikely to INCREASE deaths from melanoma because it is LOWER amounts of sunlight (and its parts) that are linked with more deaths from melanoma. Of course, this is a basic point but it is worth spelling out because the matter can seem confusing.

There is a second reason as well for the unlikelihood of the connection between indoor tanning and melanoma deaths - confound. Patrons are more likely to visit tanning places in areas where the sun is weaker. There was a tanning place where I stayed in Anchorage Alaska but not where I stayed in Honolulu Hawaii. In other words, people are more likely to visit tanning places in areas that have a higher death rate from melanoma to start with (due to the low ultraviolet in natural sunlight in those more northern, colder places). As the model shows a clearly higher death rate from melanoma in these northern places, this could be attributed mistakenly to the more frequent use of indoor tanning machines.

While any connection between indoor tanning is unlikely given the results of the model, I am not making the broader claim that such machines are safe. One example of concern is the large amount of heat given off from tanning bulbs. Not enough effort is made to adequately move this heat buildup away from the patron which might be generally unhealthy.

As for melanoma, however, even this concern is not relevant because heat is the product of infrared radiation in sunlight and it, as well, being correlated with the rest of sunlight, is unlikely to be linked with melanoma. This is because, in a separate model not shown, heat from sunlight (air temperature) is also linked with melanoma but in the OPPOSITE direction. The hotter the air over the course of the year, the fewer the deaths from melanoma in that place.

I will end with a concluding word about the difficulty of gaining an intuitive sense of a connection that is negative in direction. In this model, we found a link between ultraviolet in sunlight reaching the ground over the course of the year, and deaths from melanoma but in a direction opposite to what one might expect. LOWER yearly levels of ultraviolet reaching the ground are linked with MORE deaths from melanoma.

The human brain is able to remember who WAS at the party but has a more difficult time thinking about who was NOT there. As an example, even I have thought it plausible to change this negative connection to a positive one by coming up with two alternative possibilities. Perhaps it was exposure to ultraviolet-depleted sunlight that was responsible for melanoma. Or perhaps it was exposure to sunlight that was UVB-depleted with its higher portion of UVA that was responsible for melanoma. Neither alternative ideas performed very well as explanations for the main result.

In light of the radical nature of the research result here, we must, of course, wait for future research to see if such studies conflict with or confirm this result. The result seems far less radical in the context of the research presented here on many other cancers suggesting a similar conclusion – more deaths from cancer the weaker the ultraviolet reaching the ground becomes.

Chapter 7. Cancer of the Urinary Tract Including Bladder Cancer and a Link with Insufficiently Strong Ultraviolet in Sunlight as a Result of Living Too Far North.

Bladder cancer is part of the death category (on the Health Data Interactive site) called cancer of the urinary tract. The death rate from urinary tract cancer in 2011-2013 is 12.4 deaths per hundred thousand in the adult population (age 18 and over). The death rate from cancer in general is 241.4 deaths. This means that urinary tract cancer as a percent of all deaths from cancer is 12.4/241.4=.051 or 5.1 percent. The death rate from all causes (not just cancer) is 1047.0 so urinary tract cancer as a percent of all deaths during these years is 12.4/1047.0=.012 or 1.2 percent.

What portion of the urinary tract cancer category is specifically bladder cancer? The site Health Data Interactive is now closed (late July 2016) making it a modest challenge to answer this question. From other sources, however, we learn that bladder cancer as a percent of all cancer deaths is about 2.8 percent. Given that the broader urinary tract category is 5.1 percent of all deaths from cancer, this means that cancers of other urinary tract sites are 5.1-2.8=2.3 or about 2.3 percent of all cancer deaths. As a portion of all urinary tract cancer deaths, then, bladder cancer specifically represents 2.8/5.1=.549 or 54.9 percent, the majority of deaths in this category. The non-bladder portion of this urinary tract category represents 2.3/5.1=.451 or 45 percent of this category that we will model here. Lastly, while urinary tract cancer represents 1.2 percent of all deaths, bladder cancer specifically represents .549*1.2=.659 or .66 percent of all deaths, or a little less than seven tenths of one percent of all deaths.

This confirms an estimate from other bladder cancer numbers suggesting that deaths from bladder cancer are between a half and three quarters of one percent of all deaths in the most recent year available. While my interest is greatest in bladder cancer specifically, we must now refer to all results as the broader category of urinary tract cancer.

Of a few choices, the best numbers for producing a successful model were primarily chosen based on the highest explanatory power of the total model (Adjusted R Square). This is death rates from cancers of the urinary tract for the years 2004, 2005 and 2006.

Table 7-1 [urinry46] urinary tract cancer death rate, yearly average between 2004 and 2006, majority from bladder cancer.

Alaska	4.3	District	9.3
Utah	5.2	Michigan	9.3
Hawaii	5.8	New Hampshire	9.4
Georgia	6.6	Arkansas	9.5
Colorado	6.9	Connecticut	9.6
California	7.2	Montana	9.7
Texas	7.3	Oregon	9.7
New Mexico	7.7	Kentucky	9.8
Virginia	7.7	Indiana	9.8
Wyoming	7.8	Nebraska	10.0
Idaho	7.9	Oklahoma	10.1
Mississippi	8.2	Missouri	10.1
Maryland	8.2	Massachusetts	10.4
Arizona	8.4	Florida	10.6
South Carolina	8.4	Ohio	10.7
Alabama	8.6	Wisconsin	10.8
Nevada	8.6	Iowa	11.0
North Carolina	8.6	Delaware	11.1
New York	8.7	West Virginia	11.4
Illinois	8.8	Pennsylvania	11.4
Minnesota	8.9	Vermont	11.4
Washington	8.9	South Dakota	11.8
Louisiana	9.2	Rhode Island	11.8
New Jersey	9.2	North Dakota	12.1
Tennessee	9.3	Maine	12.4
Kansas	9.3		

This list can be found in Table 7-1 [urinry46] "Urinary tract cancer death rates by state, 2004-2006". Of course, these numbers are crude rates not adjusted by age and, therefore, are influenced by the proportion of the population that is in the older age category (65 and over).

For this reason, the lowest rate in Table 7-1 is in Alaska, 4.3 deaths per hundred thousand population. This low number is probably highly influenced by the fact that there are so few older people in Alaska, many of whom retire to warmer places, I imagine. The highest rate for urinary tract cancer is in Maine at 12.4 deaths. This difference represents nice variation, a solid two times plus from the lowest to the highest rate (using the second lowest rate for Utah at 5.2 deaths compared to the highest in Maine at 12.4 deaths).

The final model which best explains the pattern of differences between states in dying from urinary tract cancer in Table 7-1 is short and simple. It is composed of two items. The higher the percent of older people in the population of the state (age 65 and over), the higher the death rate from urinary tract cancer.

The second item is the intensity of ultraviolet reaching the ground during a multi year period from 2006-2014, a scientifically sophisticated measurement of ultraviolet based on the UV Index of NOAA. As I have mentioned in earlier chapters, this composite calculation was most kindly provided me by their scientist Craig Long for whom I feel a deep sense of gratitude. This single number of the average UV Index during this long multi-year period is some integration of daily predictions of ultraviolet reaching the ground in each of my large cities, one to represent each state (including Washington DC, which I call "District" in the list of "states").

To make this daily prediction, NOAA (similar to government agencies in various countries) uses satellite weather data, such as cloud cover and rain, to calculate the strength of ultraviolet (in sunlight) for each city. The focus is on the strength reaching the ground at the time when the sun is strongest during the day which happens to be at "solar noon". This is the time around noon or one o'clock depending on whether daylight savings time is in force. The time of solar noon is also affected by the particular location of the city within the time zone band. It varies slightly based on how east or west the city happens to be within that time zone.

A further important transformation made for constructing the UV Index (UVI) is the changing of the absolute energy of the ultraviolet in sunlight reaching the ground into a form which better captures its effect on human skin. These daily "predictions" for the UVI (UV Index) are published in the afternoon of the preceding day and are like a weather forecast for the following day. They summarize the best guess for how strong the ultraviolet will be the following day around noon in that city.

During the summer in some places, radio stations include this information in weather forecasts to help people going to the beach avoid getting sunburned. The final UV Index number is from 1 to about 12, going up to 16, I believe. It is this number that has been aggregated into a yearly average for each city for my earlier 1996 measure and a multi year average for this much more recent estimate. To my surprise, both measures are highly correlated with each other with [ultra96] and [uvi0614] having a correlation of .993.

This model for urinary tract cancer deaths in 2004-2006 is the first to "work" with the newer, multiyear, set of ultraviolet numbers. (It also appears in lung cancer Chapter 3 which was one of the last models I worked on even though it appeared as an earlier chapter in the book in light of its large size). The weaker the strength of ultraviolet reaching the ground in the largest city of the state (as you drive north in the United States), the higher the death rate from urinary tract cancer. This is the result in the full model, the details of which will following shortly.

While a bit premature to comment on the result, there is little question in my mind that this surprising result is largely due to the sophisticated science behind this unique way of capturing the strength of ultraviolet in sunlight through the use of the UV Index in aggregated form.

In keeping with the pattern here to introduce each item in the model before presenting the final model, the state list for percent age 65 is found in Table 7-2.

From the older age Table 7-2, we learn from this somewhat familiar list that the state with the lowest percent of seniors is indeed Alaska at 6.8 percent, with the highest being Florida at 16.8 percent. Thus, in Florida, the senior portion of the population is more than twice as large compared to that of Alaska. (6.8/100=16.8/x. 1680=6.8x. 1680/6.8=x. x=247.06 [or (compared to 100) about two and a half times greater].

Table 7-2 older age.
Percent of the state population that is Age 65 and Over (2006)

State	%	State	%
Alaska	6.8	New Jersey	12.9
Utah	8.8	Kansas	12.9
Georgia	9.8	Oregon	12.9
Texas	9.9	Wisconsin	13.0
Colorado	10.0	New York	13.1
California	10.8	Oklahoma	13.2
Nevada	11.1	Nebraska	13.3
Idaho	11.5	Massachusetts	13.3
Washington	11.5	Vermont	13.3
Virginia	11.6	Missouri	13.3
Maryland	11.6	Connecticut	13.4
Illinois	12.0	Delaware	13.4
Minnesota	12.1	Alabama	13.4
Wyoming	12.2	Ohio	13.4
North Carolina	12.2	Montana	13.8
Louisiana	12.2	Rhode Island	13.9
District	12.3	Arkansas	13.9
New Mexico	12.4	Hawaii	14.0
New Hampshire	12.4	South Dakota	14.2
Indiana	12.4	North Dakota	14.6
Mississippi	12.4	Iowa	14.6
Michigan	12.5	Maine	14.6
Tennessee	12.7	Pennsylvania	15.2
Arizona	12.8	West Virginia	15.3
South Carolina	12.8	Florida	16.8
Kentucky	12.8		

While is seems unexciting to learn that older age is linked with a higher death rate from bladder cancer, it is, nevertheless, important to specify in this case, mainly for technical reasons. Due to the large connection between older age and dying from various cancers, it is vitally important to account for that connection in these statistical models which are attempts to explain the pattern of deaths across states. This is because it is, to a large extent, a prerequisite for inquiring further to learn what else might help to explain the death rate pattern.

Table 7-3 is the ultraviolet list of states, ultraviolet reaching the ground as part of sunlight in the largest city of the state based on the UV Index in the form of a composite number over the nine year period of 2006-2014. It goes from a low UVI (UV Index) score of 1.9 in Alaska (Anchorage) to a high of 11.1 for Hawaii (Honolulu).

It is interesting to note that the second highest UVI is for the state of Florida (Miami) at 8.5. While still relatively high, a look at the map of the United States makes clear that, while Florida is "south", Hawaii, across the country, is much further south, closer to the equator. Thus, it is not surprising that the UV Index value is not as strong for Florida (8.5) compared to Hawaii (11.1). Of course, the value for summertime is actually higher overall by a certain amount. This is because the UVI values in Table 7-3 are a measure of sunlight (the ultraviolet part) over the course of the entire year which includes the much weaker winter sun.

Having now introduced the items in the model, we can turn to the urinary tract cancer model page in Table 7-4. As is our pattern, we start with the bottom box of individual correlations to make sure that there is no troubling connection between the items in the model (the two "independent variables" of age and ultraviolet) which could create skewed, misleading results. Thankfully, the correlation between them is small in size (.090) and not statistically significant (no stars). I call this kind of model "clean".

While we are in the bottom box of Table 7-4, we also glance at the "zero order" correlations between each item and the matter at hand, death rates from urinary tract cancer. We see connections at this early stage. Both have two stars, meaning significant at the .01 level. There is a not surprising correlation (in the bottom row) between age and urinary tract cancer death rates of .804**. Also, there is a connection between ultraviolet and urinary tract cancer of minus (-) .370**. The minus means, more ultraviolet, fewer deaths from urinary tract cancer.

Table 7-3 [uvi0614]
UVI (UV Index) between 2006 and 2014. Ultraviolet. Average annual UVI (UV Index) score over a nine year period for the largest city in the state.

State	UVI	State	UVI
Alaska	1.9	West Virginia	4.6
Washington	3.5	Kentucky	4.8
Oregon	3.6	Missouri	4.8
Vermont	3.6	Idaho	4.9
Minnesota	3.9	Kansas	5.2
North Dakota	3.9	Virginia	5.4
Maine	3.9	North Carolina	5.4
Michigan	4.0	Wyoming	5.5
New Hampshire	4.0	Tennessee	5.5
Wisconsin	4.1	Arkansas	5.6
Illinois	4.2	Oklahoma	5.6
Connecticut	4.2	Utah	5.7
Massachusetts	4.2	Colorado	5.8
Ohio	4.2	Georgia	6.0
South Dakota	4.2	South Carolina	6.3
Rhode Island	4.2	Nevada	6.3
Iowa	4.3	Mississippi	6.4
New York	4.4	Texas	6.9
Montana	4.4	Arizona	6.9
Pennsylvania	4.4	California	7.0
Indiana	4.5	New Mexico	7.0
Nebraska	4.5	Alabama	7.0
Maryland	4.6	Louisiana	7.2
New Jersey	4.6	Florida	8.5
District	4.6	Hawaii	11.1
Delaware	4.6		

Flipping this around, the weaker the ultraviolet, the more deaths from urinary tract cancer.

This result so far is rather rare because often, the interesting result only shows up in the main model above. In this case, a connection between the strength of ultraviolet and urinary tract cancer is already apparent here. To assess its strength, however, it is still best to wait for the final model.

Before discussing the final model in the middle box of Table 7-4, we can first skip to the top box to learn about the total explanatory power of the model as a whole, how good a job it does in explaining the difference between states in dying from cancer of the urinary tract. The Adjusted R Square in that top box is .838 meaning that the model explains 83.8 percent of the total pattern. In the context of these models, this is a large number suggesting a successful model.

Now we are ready to turn to the final model in the middle box (of Table 7-4). We start at the right with the statistical significance test.

Of course, as I have stated elsewhere, these numbers for urinary tract cancer deaths over the course of the three year period are no mere sample but are actually the entire population of deaths (as accurately as the recording of deaths tells us). Individual deaths from this cancer group are grouped by state and converted to a death rate per hundred thousand people. Nevertheless, whether necessary or not, I use a statistical test for these models having decided to treat these death rate lists as a hypothetical subset of a larger population of all deaths from cancers in this area of the body over time and over various places.

More informally, I use the statistical test to evaluate the solidness of the result. Furthermore, the work here uses the more stringent significance level of .01 which further adds to the impression that the resulting connection, in this case, between weaker ultraviolet and deaths from urinary tract cancer, is very solid.

In this middle box in Table 7-4, the Sig values are both .000 and while the "t" score must be larger than 2 (forgetting the sign right now), both connections are larger. The connection with age is a very large almost 15, and with ultraviolet, also a very large about 8.

Table 7-4 The model for urinary tract cancer: stronger ultraviolet, fewer deaths

Model Summary

Model	R	R Square	Adjusted R Square	Std. Error of the Estimate
1	.919[a]	.844	.838	.6978

a. Predictors: (Constant), UVI0614, AGE65IN6

Coefficients[a]

Model		Unstandardized Coefficients		Standardized Coefficients	t	Sig.
		B	Std. Error	Beta		
1	(Constant)	.796	.802		.993	.325
	AGE65IN6	.874	.059	.844	14.755	.000
	UVI0614	-.519	.067	-.446	-7.790	.000

a. Dependent Variable: URINRY46

Correlations

		AGE65IN6	UVI0614	URINRY46
AGE65IN6	Pearson Correlation	1	.090	.804**
	Sig. (2-tailed)	.	.531	.000
	N	51	51	51
UVI0614	Pearson Correlation	.090	1	-.370**
	Sig. (2-tailed)	.531	.	.008
	N	51	51	51
URINRY46	Pearson Correlation	.804**	-.370**	1
	Sig. (2-tailed)	.000	.008	.
	N	51	51	51

**. Correlation is significant at the 0.01 level (2-tailed).

Of course, other threats to validity remain. The actual connection with urinary tract cancer might not be weaker ultraviolet but rather something else correlated with weaker ultraviolet. There are many environmental items which vary with south to north latitude and we can never be entirely certain that we have picked the right one. The best we can do is test this choice against other alternatives. (These many alternative models, less successful, are not shown here as I focus only on the best result).

The purpose of the elaborate testing of various models is to bolster confidence in the belief that we have made the best choice among those tested. Our goal was to identify the relevant connection which best explained the pattern across the states in deaths from cancer of the urinary tract. In the end, all we can do is provide evidence that this connection might be the most fruitful and relevant one. The method itself, however, prevents us from ever being entirely certain. Here, we are building a case, strong overall, that something interesting is going on between ultraviolet and cancer of the urinary tract.

With the statistical tests behind us, we now move to the middle Beta column, (middle box in Table 7-4), our first look at the size of both effects on urinary tract cancer. Ignoring the decimals and the minus sign for now, we see that the age effect (844) is larger than the ultraviolet effect (446). As part of this explained portion of the pattern between states (calling this 100%), we add both numbers together (again ignoring the signs for now) 844+446=1290. Age is 844/1290=.654 or 65.4 percent of the explained portion. Ultraviolet is 466/1290=.361 or 36.1 percent of the explained portion.

We also want to know how much each item explains of the total pattern between states. Of course, as the model explains only 83.8 percent of the pattern, less that 100 percent of the possible explanation, these next numbers will be smaller.

To come up with the new denominator, we use the earlier one of 1290 which represents .838 (from the Adjusted R Square) and we want to know the number that represents 1. 1290/.838=x/1. .838x=1290. x=1290/.838=1539.38. For age now, 844/1539.38=.548. Of the total explanation of the pattern of death rates from urinary cancer between the states, older age represents 54.8 percent, a little over half. (While this IS lower than the original 65 percent, it is not lower by that much given that the model explains such a high portion of the possible explanation, about 84 percent).

For ultraviolet, it is 446/1539.38=.290 or 29 percent of the total explanation for the pattern of difference between states in dying from urinary tract cancer. So the difference between states in how strong the ultraviolet is – is linked to the death rate from urinary tract cancer. Furthermore, it explains 29 percent of this pattern across the states, more than a quarter.

Now we are finally ready for the actual equation in the B column of the middle box in Table 7-4. These are the numbers we use to write a numerical summary of the result of our attempt to best explain the set of numbers in Table 7-1, the actual death rate from urinary tract cancer across the states. Our two items explain this pattern which is best summarized in this set of numbers using the values for each state in these lists of the two items in Table 7-2 older age, and Table 7-3 ultraviolet.

We use these numbers not to try to replicate the original list in Table 7-1 as best we can but rather to construct a different list of numbers which gives us a better view of the relationship we have discovered between weaker ultraviolet and more deaths from urinary tract cancer. To construct this "best view", we use the equation in the middle box in Table 7-4 to set aside the effect of age allowing us to see more clearly the effect of ultraviolet.

We do this by plugging in the average percent in the older age category for all the states when running the equation. This happens to be 12.653 or around 13 percent. For our item of interest, ultraviolet, we use the actual value for ultraviolet strength over the time period from the ultraviolet list in Table 7-3. We can now write that equation and then run it. Using the numbers in the B column of the middle box in Table 7-4, it is as follows. .796 + (.874 * 12.653) - (.519 * uvi0614).

Running this equation yields the new list of predicted urinary tract cancer death rates in Table 7-5. I call this the "best view" because it gives us our first look at the pattern after setting aside the large effect of older age on the original death rate list in Table 7-1. For this best look list of death rates, only ultraviolet is allowed to vary.

Thus, the ordering of states in this list is identical to the list of states in the ultraviolet list in Table 7-3 but with one important difference. When ultraviolet goes DOWN in strength (as you drive north in the US), the deaths (per population size) from urinary tract cancer go UP. So comparing the two lists, the new predicted list of death rates in Table 7-5 and the ultraviolet list in Table 7-3, the ordering of states is exactly reversed.

Table 7-5 "Best view" predicted death rates from cancer of the urinary tract including bladder. Based on actual death rates in 2004-2006. The effect of older age (more deaths) is largely removed in order to see the size of the impact of more intense ultraviolet (fewer deaths). As only ultraviolet varies, the state order is the same as in Table 7-3 ultraviolet but in reverse.

State	Rate	State	Rate
Hawaii	6.1	District	9.5
Florida	7.4	Delaware	9.5
Louisiana	8.1	West Virginia	9.5
California	8.2	Indiana	9.5
New Mexico	8.2	Nebraska	9.5
Alabama	8.2	New York	9.6
Texas	8.3	Montana	9.6
Arizona	8.3	Pennsylvania	9.6
Mississippi	8.5	Iowa	9.6
South Carolina	8.6	Illinois	9.7
Nevada	8.6	Connecticut	9.7
Georgia	8.7	Massachusetts	9.7
Colorado	8.8	Ohio	9.7
Utah	8.9	South Dakota	9.7
Arkansas	8.9	Rhode Island	9.7
Oklahoma	8.9	Wisconsin	9.7
Wyoming	9.0	Michigan	9.8
Tennessee	9.0	New Hampshire	9.8
Virginia	9.1	Minnesota	9.8
North Carolina	9.1	North Dakota	9.8
Kansas	9.2	Maine	9.8
Idaho	9.3	Oregon	10.0
Kentucky	9.4	Vermont	10.0
Missouri	9.4	Washington	10.0
Maryland	9.5	Alaska	10.9
New Jersey	9.5		

On the ultraviolet list, Hawaii is the state with the strongest ultraviolet, but we learn from the "best view" list in Table 7-5 that Hawaii has the lowest "predicted" death rate from cancer of the urinary tract. Conversely, Alaska has the weakest ultraviolet reaching the ground in Table 7-3 but it has the highest predicted death rate from urinary tract cancer, at the bottom of the list in Table 7-5. (The numbers in this "best view" list in Table 7-5 are the predicted death rates based on the actual death rates in 2004-2006 from Table 7-1. They are based on the equation we developed from our attempt to explain that pattern of numbers in Table 7-1).

By moving the large matter of older age to the side, we now have a chance in Table 7-5 to see the size of the effect of ultraviolet on urinary tract cancer death rates. To figure out the size of the effect of ultraviolet on death rates from cancer of the urinary tract, we know that the rate (in Table 7-5) is lowest at 6.1 deaths per hundred thousand people in the highest UV state of Hawaii and highest in Alaska (10.9 deaths) in the lowest UV state, the state with the weakest ultraviolet reaching the ground over the course of the year. Compared with the lowest death rate state (set at 100), the urinary tract cancer death rate in the highest death rate state is 178.7 or 78.7 percent larger in size. (6.1/100=10.9/x. 1090=6.1x. x=1090/6.1. x=178.7).

In other words, due to the effect of too-weak ultraviolet reaching the ground, the death rate from this cancer can go up a maximum of 78.7 percent. More generally, compared to the state with the strongest ultraviolet, the state with the weakest ultraviolet has a death rate from urinary tract cancer that is 78.7 percent higher, higher by some three quarters.

As best as we can tell, that difference is due to how weak the sun is (its ultraviolet portion). The weaker the sun's ultraviolet, the more people die from urinary tract cancer. In fact, due to weaker ultraviolet, the death rate almost doubles, going up by some three quarters. For the first time here (as I wrote this chapter early), I figured out that this "best view" list of death rates can sometimes be used to give another view of the size of the effect of interest, in this case, ultraviolet.

How can we interpret the main finding of interest here, that weak ultraviolet is linked with more deaths from urinary tract cancer, a death category that includes cancer of the bladder? It should be clear that this coming part of the analysis is speculation for a series of reasons. First, I suspect that nobody knows for sure why weaker ultraviolet in sunlight is linked with more deaths from urinary tract cancer. Furthermore, I am not trained as a medical doctor, or an oncologist, or a cell biologist or a geneticist. On the other hand, while this specific finding with urinary tract cancer is entirely new, I have actually had nineteen years to speculate about this question having found hints about this general result in previous work (even though the finding for bladder cancer specifically is only days old).

My best guess is that ultraviolet stimulates travel through the cell cycle, speeding the process of cell replication. It is this speeding up of the cell cycle that somehow prevent cells turning to cancer (however contrarian the notion given that cancer is out-of-control replication). To prevent cancer in this part of the body, the urinary tract, it is possible that some exposure to strong enough ultraviolet in sunlight might prevent the cell cycle from stalling.

The relationship uncovered in the model here between weaker ultraviolet and more deaths from urinary tract cancer is linear in nature, with a unit decrease in ultraviolet linked to a unit increase in deaths from this group of cancers. Nevertheless, I wonder if there is a certain threshold of strength of the sunlight reaching the ground in order for sunlight to work to stimulate its posited therapeutic effect on the cell cycle. In many places, sunlight and its ultraviolet might simply be too weak to effectively play this posited therapeutic role.

If such is the case, then why does not everybody in Alaska get bladder cancer and die of it (God forbid)? I do not know. This model explains only the difference in death rates between places. It cannot well explain the difference between outcomes in the same location, the same city – why one person dies of it and the other not. Here, perhaps, different patterns of outdoor exposure to sunlight and whether such exposure includes the midday sun when ultraviolet is highest during the day, might also play a role.

At best, "exposure" to sunlight as an explanation of these differences between states in deaths from urinary tract cancer would only partly explain the ultraviolet finding here. While it might be the case that people spend more time outdoors in sunnier places, this seems incomplete as a satisfying explanation for the ultraviolet finding here.

People typically work in offices during the day regardless of how nice the weather is outside. This is why I return to the actual strength of sunlight and its ultraviolet reaching the ground as perhaps a more likely explanation for the difference between places. While "exposure" to sunlight might or might not be different in different parts of the country related to the weather, this would not make much difference if the sunlight (and its ultraviolet) is not strong enough in the first place to have its posited therapeutic effect.

Chapter 8. Non-Hodgkin's Lymphoma and a link with the Earth's Stronger Magnetic Field as We Drive North (in the United States)

This chapter deals exclusively with dying from non-Hodgkin's lymphoma but I usually refer to it here as simply lymphoma. In the period 2011-2013, the yearly death rate for the entire United States from Non-Hodgkin's Lymphoma was 8.4 deaths per hundred thousand people. All deaths from cancer during these years (annual) was 241.4 deaths per hundred thousand, and deaths from all causes was 1047.0. Lymphoma as a portion of all deaths from cancer is 8.4/241.4=.0347 or about 3.5 percent (of all deaths from cancer). Lymphoma as a percent of deaths from all causes is 8.4/1047.0=.0080 or .8 percent of all deaths (eight tenth of one percent, a little less than one percent).

In Table 8-1, we find death rates from lymphoma by state for the years 2004-2006 on an annual basis. Above, the death rate percents are for later years for purposes of comparison with other cancers.

For this cancer, I selected an earlier set of years because the model test was much better based on Adjusted R Square, due, I suspect, to mistakes in the 2011-2013 numbers. This is just a guess, however. The more successful list from these earlier years provided a better way for testing various possible combinations of items with the goal of building the best explanation possible here for dying from lymphoma.

As usual, we begin with the actual death rate list for lymphoma in Table 8-1: Lymphoma: Non-Hodgkin's lymphoma death rates by state 2004-2006. Alaska has the lowest annual death rate of 2.5 deaths while Pennsylvania has the highest of 9.4 deaths. Alaska looks like an "outlier", unusually low, perhaps partly because of how few seniors live in such a cold state (Table 8-2). This low death rate still seems unusual given that lymphoma is linked with higher Earth magnetism (Table 8-3). We would expect the strength of ground level geomagnetism to be relatively high in Alaska due to its northern location (Table 8-3). It turns out, however, that it is not as high as we would expect, coming in at 14 highest (out of 51).

Back to the death rates in Table 8-1, it is helpful to get a sense of the spread between states. Compared with Alaska, the death rate in Pennsylvania, the highest state, is considerably higher. It is useful to figure out by how much. 3.5/100=9.4/x. 3.5x=940. x=940/3.5. x=268.6. The lymphoma death rate in the highest state (compared to the lowest) is well over twice as high, some two and two thirds times higher (almost three times higher).

Table 8-1 Lymphoma:
Non-Hodgkin's lymphoma death rates by state 2004-2006

State	Rate	State	Rate
Alaska	3.5	Oklahoma	7.4
Utah	5.2	District	7.5
Colorado	5.2	Missouri	7.5
Georgia	5.3	Arkansas	7.6
Nevada	5.4	Kansas	7.6
New Mexico	5.4	Connecticut	7.6
Texas	5.6	Minnesota	7.6
California	5.8	Kentucky	7.7
Hawaii	5.9	Indiana	7.8
Mississippi	5.9	Ohio	7.8
Virginia	6.1	Michigan	7.8
Maryland	6.2	Tennessee	7.9
New Hampshire	6.3	Rhode Island	7.9
Arizona	6.5	Montana	7.9
South Carolina	6.5	Nebraska	8.1
Idaho	6.6	Oregon	8.2
North Carolina	6.8	Massachusetts	8.2
Vermont	6.8	Wisconsin	8.2
New York	6.9	South Dakota	8.2
Wyoming	6.9	Maine	8.5
Louisiana	7.1	Florida	8.6
Alabama	7.1	Iowa	8.7
Delaware	7.1	North Dakota	8.9
Washington	7.1	West Virginia	9.3
Illinois	7.1	Pennsylvania	9.4
New Jersey	7.3		

There are two items that explain the pattern of deaths from lymphoma across the states. The first is older age which can be found in Table 8-2 Age. Percent age 65 and over in a state (2006). The lowest percent seniors in a state is Alaska at about 7 percent while the highest percent seniors is in Florida at about 17 percent. The higher the percent seniors, the more deaths from lymphoma. This link between older age and lymphoma is both solid and large in size.

The second item which explains the pattern of deaths from lymphoma is Earth magnetism. The strength of Earth magnetism for each state can be found in Table 8-3 Magnetic. Earth Magnetism on the ground in the largest city of the state.

This particular set of numbers for Earth magnetism worked best, called [magnetic] in the upcoming model. It is an earlier measure perhaps from the late 1990s constructed by employing another calculator entering geographic characteristics of my 51 largest cities, one in each state, used to represent the state. At that time, the calculator was kindly sent to me on floppy disc (!) by a scientist at the USGS (that I recall). These numbers are not actual measurements on the ground in each location but are rather based on a model of the estimated geomagnetic field strength on the ground in that location.

The correlation between this earlier measure for Earth magnetism [magnetic] and another used in other models called [geomag08] is .961**. I selected this particular set of numbers because it "works better", beating out the other one in a head to head test. These numbers are an estimate of typical geomagnetic field strength on the ground in the largest city of the state measured in very small increments of nanoTeslas, nT. [1 nanoTesla is one billionth of a Tesla which also equals .01 milligauss (.01 mG)]. The size of this naturally occurring Earth magnetism is many times smaller than a child's home magnet.

Looking at Table 8-3, the lowest size of the magnetic field on the ground is in Hawaii (Honolulu) at about 36000 nT. This compares to the state with the highest ground level Earth magnetism, North Dakota at about 58000 nT.

Compared to the lowest reading in Hawaii, the reading in North Dakota is larger by an amount we can now calculate.   35625.4/100=58249.5/x. 35625.4x=4824950. x=4824950/35625.4. x=135.44. The highest reading is thus about 35% higher than the lowest reading (among US states).

Table 8-2 Age. Percent age 65 and over in a state (2006)

State	%	State	%
Alaska	6.8	New Jersey	12.9
Utah	8.8	Kansas	12.9
Georgia	9.8	Oregon	12.9
Texas	9.9	Wisconsin	13.0
Colorado	10.0	New York	13.1
California	10.8	Oklahoma	13.2
Nevada	11.1	Vermont	13.3
Idaho	11.5	Missouri	13.3
Washington	11.5	Nebraska	13.3
Virginia	11.6	Massachusetts	13.3
Maryland	11.6	Alabama	13.4
Illinois	12.0	Delaware	13.4
Minnesota	12.1	Connecticut	13.4
North Carolina	12.2	Ohio	13.4
Wyoming	12.2	Montana	13.8
Louisiana	12.2	Arkansas	13.9
District	12.3	Rhode Island	13.9
New Mexico	12.4	Hawaii	14.0
Mississippi	12.4	South Dakota	14.2
New Hampshire	12.4	Maine	14.6
Indiana	12.4	Iowa	14.6
Michigan	12.5	North Dakota	14.6
Tennessee	12.7	Pennsylvania	15.2
Arizona	12.8	West Virginia	15.3
South Carolina	12.8	Florida	16.8
Kentucky	12.8		

Table 8-3 Magnetic.
Earth Magnetism on the ground in the largest city of the state

Hawaii	35625.4	Rhode Island	54405.8
Florida	46661.5	Oregon	54488.2
California	48806.5	Colorado	54495.4
Texas	49535.4	Massachusetts	54569.3
Arizona	49659.1	Kentucky	54602.1
Louisiana	49840.3	Connecticut	54625.9
Alabama	50301.8	Idaho	54747.8
Nevada	50726.3	Missouri	54943.7
South Carolina	51040.2	Maine	54957.6
Mississippi	51318.5	New Hampshire	55023.4
New Mexico	51567.1	Wyoming	55245.4
Georgia	52012.6	Alaska	55332.5
North Carolina	52601.4	Indiana	55391.8
Arkansas	52766.1	Washington	55578.2
Virginia	52847.1	Ohio	55844.2
Oklahoma	52918.3	Vermont	55849.6
Tennessee	53024.6	Nebraska	56143.5
New Jersey	53819.1	Michigan	56346.6
Utah	53981.5	Iowa	56382.3
District	54012.4	Illinois	56456.8
Maryland	54145.9	Wisconsin	56977.3
Delaware	54195.8	Montana	57023.5
Kansas	54198.2	South Dakota	57158.0
Pennsylvania	54228.3	Minnesota	57859.2
West Virginia	54322.4	North Dakota	58249.5
New York	54404.6		

Now that we are somewhat familiar with the items in the lymphoma model, we can view the model explaining the pattern of deaths from lymphoma in Table 8-4. First we skip to the bottom box to check correlations mainly to make sure that the items fulfill a requirement of the method, that they be as little related to each other as is possible. We can see that both items are not significantly linked with each other, age 65 and magnetic. I call this result "clean".

Next is the zero order correlation with what interests us, lymphoma, in the bottom line. This is an extra, interesting even though not essential. We see the very strong connection between age and lymphoma as the correlation is .842**. Dying from lymphoma is strongly linked with the age 65 plus age category. The zero order correlation also reveals that there is little discernible connection between Earth magnetism and lymphoma (.341*)(not two stars). Apparently, this connection will only reveal itself in the full model after we have accounted for the connection with age.

Now we are ready to proceed to the actual model in Table 8-4. We move to the top box with the Adjusted R Square of .837. This gives us an idea about how well the model did in explaining the pattern of deaths from lymphoma across all of the states. The model explains 83.7 percent of the pattern, which sounds pretty high. We will soon see that most of this explanation is due to the less exciting result that older people are probably more likely to die from this disease. We already know that older people are more likely to get cancer and die from it, as well as to die in general.

We now turn to the actual lymphoma model in the middle box in Table 8-4. Starting on the right, we see the two boxes which tell us about statistical significance, how solid the result is for inferring to a broader population, for example, deaths from lymphoma in other sets of years. The result suggests that the model is solid with a Sig. value of .000 for both items. "t" is well over the required 2 value with the connection between lymphoma and age showing a value of near 15. The connection between lymphoma and Earth magnetism [magnetic] shows a t value of 6.

Table 8-4 The Non-Hodgkins Lymphoma model.
The role of stronger Earth Magnetism (more deaths).

Model Summary

Model	R	R Square	Adjusted R Square	Std. Error of the Estimate
1	.918[a]	.843	.837	.4810

a. Predictors: (Constant), MAGNETIC, AGE65IN6

Coefficients[a]

Model		Unstandardized Coefficients		Standardized Coefficients	t	Sig.
		B	Std. Error	Beta		
1	(Constant)	-7.154	1.168		-6.125	.000
	AGE65IN6	.607	.041	.853	14.918	.000
	MAGNETIC	1.232E-04	.000	.366	6.398	.000

a. Dependent Variable: LYMPH46

Correlations

		AGE65IN6	MAGNETIC	LYMPH46
AGE65IN6	Pearson Correlation	1	-.029	.842**
	Sig. (2-tailed)	.	.839	.000
	N	51	51	51
MAGNETIC	Pearson Correlation	-.029	1	.341*
	Sig. (2-tailed)	.839	.	.014
	N	51	51	51
LYMPH46	Pearson Correlation	.842*	.341*	1
	Sig. (2-tailed)	.000	.014	.
	N	51	51	51

**. Correlation is significant at the 0.01 level (2-tailed).
*. Correlation is significant at the 0.05 level (2-tailed).

The Beta column allows us to assess the relative and absolute size of these effects for explaining the pattern of deaths from lymphoma between states. These numbers can be compared directly to each other. It is clear that age is the larger effect. If we add these numbers together and divide each by that total, we get the relative effect that each contributes to the model's explanation. Excluding the decimals and signs (not relevant here), this is 853+366=1219. 853/1219=.70. Age explains 70 percent of the pattern captured by the model. 366/1219=.30. Earth magnetism [magnetic] explains about 30 percent of the pattern explained by the model. These two numbers should, of course, add to 100% which they do.

More interesting, perhaps, is knowing the absolute size of each effect as part of the total explanation for the pattern between states. We know from the Adjusted R Square that we have only succeeded in explaining part of the pattern between states, albeit a large part (about 84%). For this, we need a new denominator knowing that the sum of the two items adds to 1219 but that this is only .837 of the total pattern. 1219/.837=x/1. 1219=.837x. x=1219/.837. x=1456.39, our new denominator.

First is age. 853/1456.39=.5857. For the total pattern between states, older age accounts for 58.57 percent or about 59 percent. Now magnetism. 366/1456.39=.25. The size of the Earth's magnetic field in the largest city of the state accounts for 25 percent of the total pattern of differences between the states in deaths from lymphoma. A quarter of the pattern of dying from lymphoma can be explained by the link with geomagnetic field strength, the strength of the Earth's magnetic field on the ground in the largest city of the state. (According to this pattern, the more north we drive, the higher the strength of Earth magnetism and the more people die from lymphoma).

We are ready now to move to the B column in the middle box with the lymphoma model where we see the actual numbers of the equation. These numbers are a concise way of summarizing the model result as an equation. This equation is our best attempt to explain the pattern of lymphoma deaths across all of the states in Table 8-1. While not necessary, I convert the number for [magnetic] to the more familiar form of .0001232. We will now use these numbers, this equation, to get a better view of the pattern of deaths from lymphoma across the states than the original one in Table 8-1 (clouded due to the big impact of older age. But "percent seniors" varies from state to state).

We can do this by "controlling for" age. Of course, we are more interested to see the pattern of deaths after taking into consideration the obvious fact that there is a link between older age and dying from lymphoma. We can do this by instructing the (statistical software) program NOT to use the actual age numbers in Table 8-2 but instead to plug in one number, the average age for all the states, the mean, which happens to be 12.653. (The average percent seniors in all the states is about 13 percent).

For magnetism, however, what really interests us, we instruct the program to use the actual values in Table 8-3 for each state. We will do this now to yield a list of predicted death rates from lymphoma after zeroing out the impact of older age to see the effect that the other item has on deaths from lymphoma.

Here this other item is Earth magnetism. As this is the only item to vary, the ordering of the states will be identical to the ordering of the states in the magnetic list Table 8-3. By using the actual equation representing the real list of death rates in Table 8-1, we will end up with new death rate numbers after accounting for the effect of older age.

In SPSS 11, from the data file, we pull down "transform" and then highlight "compute". We can call this item (with our 8 character maximum) lymphmag (lymphoma magnetic). Using the numbers from the B column now, we have lymphmag = -7.154 + (.607 * 12.653) + (.0001232 * magnetic).

We find the result in Table 8-5 lymphmag (lymphoma magnetic): Best View predicted death rates from lymphoma based on actual death rates in 2004-2006 after accounting for the effect of older age (more deaths). Earth magnetism is allowed to vary while older age remains constant.

Looking now at Table 8-5, the lowest death rate state for lymphoma is now Hawaii at about 5 deaths (per hundred thousand people) and the highest is North Dakota at about 8 deaths. Now we want to find out how much higher the death rate is in the highest state compared with the lowest death rate state. 4.92/100=7.70/x. 4.92x=770. x=770/4.92. x=156.5. This estimated lymphoma death rate in the highest state, North Dakota (compared to the lowest, Hawaii) is 56.5 percent greater, over fifty percent. This view, after accounting for the effect of older age, is another way of showing the size of the effect of Earth magnetism on the pattern of deaths from lymphoma across the country.

Why might differences in the size of the naturally occurring magnetic field of the Earth be involved with the pattern of dying from lymphoma (with a larger size of this field linked with more deaths)? I do not have a clear idea.

Table 8-5 lymphmag lymphoma magnetic. Best view predicted death rates from lymphoma after accounting for the effect of older age (more deaths) in order to see the impact of stronger Earth magnetism (more deaths) as we move north. As Earth magnetism is the only item to vary, the list here has the same ordering of states as in Table 8-3 Magnetic

State	Value	State	Value
Hawaii	4.92	Rhode Island	7.23
Florida	6.28	Oregon	7.24
California	6.54	Colorado	7.24
Texas	6.63	Massachusetts	7.25
Arizona	6.64	Kentucky	7.25
Louisiana	6.67	Connecticut	7.26
Alabama	6.72	Idaho	7.27
Nevada	6.78	Missouri	7.30
South Carolina	6.81	Maine	7.30
Mississippi	6.85	New Hampshire	7.31
New Mexico	6.88	Wyoming	7.33
Georgia	6.93	Alaska	7.34
North Carolina	7.01	Indiana	7.35
Arkansas	7.03	Washington	7.37
Virginia	7.04	Ohio	7.41
Oklahoma	7.05	Vermont	7.41
Tennessee	7.06	Nebraska	7.44
New Jersey	7.16	Michigan	7.47
Utah	7.18	Iowa	7.47
District	7.18	Illinois	7.48
Maryland	7.20	Wisconsin	7.55
Delaware	7.20	Montana	7.55
Kansas	7.20	South Dakota	7.57
Pennsylvania	7.21	Minnesota	7.65
West Virginia	7.22	North Dakota	7.70
New York	7.23		

It is unlikely that this result has much relevance for the proposition that "man-made" electricity is cancer-causing including power grids and the transfer of electricity as well as home wiring and appliances. All of these sources of electricity give off magnetic fields when the electricity is moving. Over the years, I looked through this literature and found it to be generally weak in terms of finding a persuasive link with cancer.

Human use of electricity involves fields that are almost entirely AC voltage (Alternating Current) which probably has a different biological effect. In contrast, Earth magnetism, is basically DC voltage, Direct Current (even though it does technically alternate over an extended period of time). The exception to this is electric motors which might have a DC magnetic component. Even here, however, I suspect that the small size of natural Earth magnetism would make the finding here not applicable to the question of whether certain electric motors would be linked with cancer such as lymphoma.

Once again, I feel a disappointment for being unable to come up with any plausible mechanism linking Earth magnetism to the development of lymphoma cancer and eventual death from the same. As one person, I am unable to come up with a complete answer for why people die from lymphoma but this need not stop me from uncovering part of the puzzle. Perhaps others might be able to take this new information and develop it into a more satisfying explanation. (In a later chapter, I do present a different twist on this lymphoma result. This was much later in chronological time, however, as the work here slowly unfolded).

Chapter 9. Pancreatic Cancer and a Link with Drinking Wine

The estimate for the number of people in the United States who would die in the year 2015 of pancreatic cancer was 40,560 (made in advance, obviously). This is a larger number than I thought. My uncle died of this cancer, may he rest in peace, as did my professor, head of my dissertation committee, of blessed memory, as well as my dear friend's mother. It is well known that death comes very quickly from time of diagnosis, usually within months, perhaps because there are few symptoms in advance.

Looking now at a listing of new cases compared with actual deaths from pancreatic cancer, both lines are slightly farther apart in recent years but they are still very close together. Decades ago, the word cancer was so feared because it was largely the equivalent of a death sentence. While not necessarily true today, for this cancer, it is still the case. For the years 2005-2011, of those diagnosed with pancreatic cancer, only 7.2 percent were still alive five years after diagnosis. In a rare bout of emotionalism, this cancer is making me feel sad.

Death numbers for this cancer by state are more difficult to find as this cancer is not one included in my main source for cancer death rates from the CDC web site. For this cancer, based on the strength of the results, I have decided to select as a final model state death rates among women only (average annual) for the years 1996-2000. The death rate list is called [panwim60], the 60 being shorthand for the last number of the beginning and ending years 1996-2000.

For purposes of comparison with other cancers, I will construct average death rates from my lists for both women and men during those years by finding the average of all the states, the mean. For [panwim06], the mean is 9.108, around 9 deaths. For [panmen06], pancreatic cancer among men, the mean is 12.347, around 12 deaths among men, a little higher number. Assuming the population is composed of about half women and half men, I think I would add both numbers together to get a total death rate (average annual for those years): 9.108+12.347=21.455. The estimated death rate for pancreatic cancer is thus about 21.5 deaths per hundred thousand people. (I am uncertain about this calculation here).

We will use the total death rates from all kinds of cancer and from all causes from the more recent years of 2009-2011 as we have done until now keeping in mind that this introduces error into the results. In the more recent years, the death rate from all kinds of cancer is 241.4 and the death rate from all causes is 1047.0. Pancreatic cancer as a rough percent of all cancer deaths is thus 21.455/241.4=.089 or 8.9 percent or about 9 percent. Substantial. Death rates from pancreatic cancer as a percent of all deaths is 21.455/1047.0=.02 or some 2 percent of all deaths.

The state death rate list for pancreatic cancer can now be found in Table 9-1: Pancreas. Death rates by state from pancreatic cancer among women (average annual) during the years 1996-2000. While I failed to write this down at the time, I just discovered that these numbers are age-adjusted (to the 2000 population).

I realized it in this way. I learned reading about pancreatic cancer that deaths go up steeply and dramatically with advancing age but yet, when I tried my age measures, percent age 65 and over [age65in6] and percent age 85 and over [p85in06], there was no significant connection in the model. I looked back at the original source and found that these numbers were, indeed, age adjusted. This is in contrast to the other cancers where I use numbers from the column "age 18 plus (crude)". I prefer doing models using numbers before they have been adjusted for age but I was happy to find any numbers for pancreatic cancer.

While I use the list in Table 9-1 Pancreas women, I thought it might be a good idea, nevertheless, to include the death numbers for men as well, which can be found in Table 9-2. I thought some people might find it interesting. Right away, we see, looking at Table 9-2 Pancreas men, that death rates among men are substantially higher. I considered merging the lists for women and men together but decided that it would introduce too much error. The concern was that this merging would foil the validity of the project entirely.

We aim to have the most pristine, error free, starting list that we are able to find in order to come up with valid results. To repeat, I chose to model "women" because the model results were strongest and hence, provided the best vehicle for testing the many items I tried, in order to see whether there was a connection with pancreatic cancer.

In one last test now, I will compare the final model using first women and then men. The model for women explains 53.2 percent of the pattern (from the Adjusted R Square) and the same model for men explains 51.2 percent of the pattern, much closer than I figured.

Table 9-1 [panwim60] pancreatic women 1996-2000.
Average yearly death rate from pancreatic
cancer among women 1996-2000

State	Rate	State	Rate
Utah	6.5	Hawaii	9.2
Montana	7.6	Arkansas	9.2
West Virginia	7.9	Tennessee	9.2
Arizona	8.0	Missouri	9.2
Idaho	8.0	North Dakota	9.2
Nebraska	8.1	Nevada	9.3
Oklahoma	8.4	Vermont	9.3
Wyoming	8.4	Alabama	9.4
Colorado	8.5	Maryland	9.5
Iowa	8.5	Maine	9.5
South Dakota	8.5	Rhode Island	9.6
Kansas	8.6	Oregon	9.6
Florida	8.7	New Hampshire	9.6
New Mexico	8.7	Michigan	9.7
Kentucky	8.7	Mississippi	9.8
Texas	8.8	Alaska	9.8
Indiana	8.8	Washington	9.8
California	9.0	Illinois	9.8
Delaware	9.0	New York	9.9
Wisconsin	9.0	Massachusetts	9.9
Georgia	9.1	Connecticut	9.9
North Carolina	9.1	New Jersey	10.1
Virginia	9.1	Louisiana	10.4
Pennsylvania	9.1	South Carolina	10.4
Ohio	9.1	District	10.9
Minnesota	9.1		

Nevertheless, I will stick with the decision to model deaths among women as the best choice in this situation.

Now we are ready to begin in earnest starting with a look at the actual death rates for women from pancreatic cancer in Table 9-1: Pancreas women. Death rates by state from pancreatic cancer among women (average annual) during the years 1996-2000. This listing of deaths is per hundred thousand people, of course. The lowest death rate state is Utah with 6.5 deaths. The highest is "District" (Washington DC) with 10.9 deaths (per hundred thousand). Compared with the lowest state, pancreatic cancer death rates in the highest state is higher by this much. 6.5/100=10.9/x.   6.5x=1090.   x=1090/6.5. x=167.7. The highest death rate state for pancreatic cancer among women is 67.7 percent higher or about two thirds higher.

In passing, we can glance over the death rate for men now in Table 9-2 noticing that more men die from this cancer and that the listing of states, while similar, is not exactly the same.

There are two items in the final model for pancreatic cancer (women). The first connection is with elevation. The lower down the place, based on the average altitude of the state, the more deaths from pancreatic cancer. The second connection is with drinking wine (all colors together). The more wine, the more deaths from pancreatic cancer.

The first item can be found in Table 9-3: State Altitude in feet (average across entire state). The second item can be found in Table 9-4 Wine Drinking. Yearly average consumption of wine per person in a state.

While this measure for wine drinking works well in the model (as we shall soon see), the list would seem to be a problem. This is because the three top wine drinking states might include drinking by visitors or outsiders as part of the total. For "District" (Washington DC), based on my stereotype perhaps, I presume it is it the free flowing alcohol at government functions and diplomatic parties. In Nevada, it is the literally free alcohol served in Las Vegas casinos and drunk by visiting tourists. (This might now have changed).   For New Hampshire, it is the swift business in their state stores (which I once visited) where low prices bring visitors from Canada as well as neighboring states across the border to save money. While I made one attempt to adjust for the New Hampshire situation, I found that it made virtually no difference and it is best to simply accept the imperfections in the list.

Table 9-2 [panmen60] pancreatic men 1996-2000.
Death rate from pancreatic cancer among men, average annual, between 1996 and 2000. Not used for the model).

State	Rate	State	Rate
Utah	9.6	Kentucky	12.4
Idaho	10.2	Georgia	12.4
Wyoming	10.2	Pennsylvania	12.6
North Dakota	10.6	New Jersey	12.6
Arizona	10.7	Indiana	12.7
New Mexico	11.0	Delaware	12.7
Oregon	11.0	North Carolina	12.7
California	11.3	Virginia	12.7
Nevada	11.3	Massachusetts	12.7
Nebraska	11.4	Arkansas	12.8
Florida	11.4	Illinois	12.8
Hawaii	11.5	Connecticut	12.9
Oklahoma	11.7	Alabama	13.0
Missouri	11.7	Maine	13.0
Montana	11.8	Alaska	13.1
West Virginia	11.8	New York	13.1
Iowa	11.9	Maryland	13.3
Ohio	11.9	South Carolina	13.3
Washington	11.9	Tennessee	13.5
Kansas	12.0	New Hampshire	13.6
Texas	12.0	Rhode Island	14.1
Wisconsin	12.0	Mississippi	14.3
Colorado	12.1	Vermont	14.4
South Dakota	12.1	Louisiana	15.4
Michigan	12.2	District	16.0
Minnesota	12.3		

Table 9-3 [altstate] altitude of state.
State altitude in feet (averaged across the entire state).

State	Altitude	State	Altitude
Delaware	60	New Hampshire	1000
Florida	100	Vermont	1000
Louisiana	100	Iowa	1100
District	150	Pennsylvania	1100
Illinois	183	Minnesota	1200
Rhode Island	200	Oklahoma	1300
New Jersey	250	West Virginia	1500
Mississippi	300	Washington	1700
Wisconsin	320	Texas	1700
Maryland	350	North Dakota	1900
South Carolina	350	Alaska	1900
Massachusetts	500	Kansas	2000
Connecticut	500	South Dakota	2200
Alabama	500	Nebraska	2600
Georgia	600	California	2900
Maine	600	Hawaii	3030
Arkansas	650	Oregon	3300
Indiana	700	Montana	3400
North Carolina	700	Arizona	4100
Kentucky	750	Idaho	5000
Missouri	800	Nevada	5500
Ohio	850	New Mexico	5700
Michigan	900	Utah	6100
Tennessee	900	Wyoming	6700
Virginia	950	Colorado	6800
New York	1000		

Table 9-4 [ethpcwyn] ethanol per capita wine.
Per person consumption of wine (all colors) based on alcohol content.

Mississippi	.09	Minnesota	.27
West Virginia	.09	Maryland	.29
Utah	.11	Montana	.29
Arkansas	.12	Virginia	.30
Iowa	.12	Maine	.33
Oklahoma	.12	Arizona	.33
Kentucky	.13	Illinois	.35
North Dakota	.13	Alaska	.36
South Dakota	.13	Idaho	.36
Kansas	.14	New York	.38
Alabama	.15	Hawaii	.38
Tennessee	.16	Florida	.39
Wyoming	.17	Colorado	.39
Ohio	.18	New Jersey	.43
Nebraska	.18	Washington	.43
South Carolina	.19	Oregon	.45
Indiana	.19	Rhode Island	.46
Pennsylvania	.20	Delaware	.47
Texas	.20	Vermont	.47
Missouri	.22	Connecticut	.49
Michigan	.22	Massachusetts	.50
Louisiana	.23	California	.50
North Carolina	.24	New Hampshire	.55
New Mexico	.24	Nevada	.62
Georgia	.25	District	.79
Wisconsin	.26		

Returning first to state altitude, I was surprised to find that altitude (elevation) of the entire state works better generally as an item predicting death rates than other ways for measuring the height of a place including both altitude of the largest city as well as changing barometric pressure at a particular elevation. While I am unsure why this is so, perhaps the average altitude of the entire state does a better job in capturing the elevation of all the state's inhabitants.

For wine drinking (Table 9-4), much can be said. Most importantly, a connection between the consumption of alcohol and pancreatic cancer has already been noted elsewhere. Here I found the strongest connection with drinking wine specifically. I have many lists for measuring the consumption of alcohol per person in a state, for drinking alcohol in general, as well as multiple measures for drinking specific kinds of alcohol including spirits (hard liquor), beer and wine.

Unfortunately, I have no measures specifically breaking down wine drinking by color and this item as well includes red, white and blush wine together. A 2014 article about the wine preference of American suggests that about 60 percent prefer red wine and 40 percent prefer white. For comparison, globally, about 55 percent drink red.

I also have measures for what I call heavy drinking, what others call "binge drinking" defined as four, five or more drinks during one social occasion. Despite trying these many ways to represent drinking alcohol, it is the list in Table 9-4 wine drinking, that works best as being connected with the pattern of deaths among women from pancreatic cancer in Table 9-1.

Does this mean that only wine is linked with dying from pancreatic cancer (and not other kinds of alcohol)? Unfortunately, I cannot say with certainty that such is the case because it is possible to build a different model, not as strong overall, with a more general way to measure alcohol consumption called alcohol per capita [alprcap]. This item includes drinking of all kinds of alcohol together. When pitted against this strongest measure for wine drinking, it "loses", falls out of the model.

Table 9-5 [alcprcap] alcohol per capita.

Alcohol consumption of all kinds per person in a state. Unit is gallons of pure enthanol consumed over the course of the year per person. (Not included in the model because it "falls out" in competition with the more strongly linked "wine drinking" item.

Utah	1.57		Georgia	2.46
West Virginia	1.81		Rhode Island	2.50
Kansas	1.94		Oregon	2.53
Kentucky	1.95		South Dakota	2.54
Oklahoma	2.01		Massachusetts	2.58
Arkansas	2.03		Texas	2.60
Pennsylvania	2.08		Illinois	2.60
Alabama	2.09		Vermont	2.62
Tennessee	2.10		South Carolina	2.64
New York	2.11		Minnesota	2.65
Iowa	2.12		Hawaii	2.66
Virginia	2.12		North Dakota	2.74
Indiana	2.14		Montana	2.74
Ohio	2.17		Wyoming	2.75
North Carolina	2.17		New Mexico	2.76
Maryland	2.28		Louisiana	2.84
Idaho	2.31		Florida	2.84
Connecticut	2.34		Colorado	2.94
Michigan	2.37		Arizona	2.94
Missouri	2.38		Wisconsin	2.98
Washington	2.39		Delaware	2.99
Mississippi	2.43		Alaska	3.00
Nebraska	2.43		District	3.97
New Jersey	2.43		New Hampshire	4.55
Maine	2.44		Nevada	4.57
California	2.45			

Clearly, wine drinking is most strongly connected with deaths from pancreatic cancer, perhaps the first finding to highlight this specific link. Perhaps I will now add alcohol per capita [alcprcap] as Table 9-5 for purposes of comparison with wine drinking in Table 9-4 because it also works in a model not shown (linked with pancreatic cancer but not as strongly, apparently). (To repeat, this broader measure for drinking alcohol falls out of the final model and is merely an extra).

Now that we are familiar with the items in the pancreatic cancer model (together with two related items that are not in this final model), we can now turn to the pancreatic cancer model itself in Table 9-6. In the top box, we see that the Adjusted R Square is .532. This model all together explains 53.2 percent of the pattern of the list of state pancreatic cancer death rates in Table 9-1.

At first glance, this Adjusted R Square number seems low compared to models for many of the other cancers. As a belated thought, however, many months after writing the original version of this chapter, I realized that such is not the case, that this result is actually strong. This is because the numbers are already adjusted for "age" which is often a large part of the Adjusted R Square value in other models.

For purposes of comparison, we can look at lymphoma whose original numbers are "crude" before any age adjustment. The effect of older age accounted for 59 percent of the total possible explanation for that cancer. While this might be, admittedly, on the high side, we can use this information to show a possible effect for older age for this cancer, however imperfect the attempt to compare two sets of death numbers, one "crude" and one already age-adjusted like the numbers here for pancreatic.

If this model of numbers here, already age-adjusted, accounts for some 54 percent of the total possible pattern, we could add the 59 percent size of the effect of age from the other cancer which would add to a sum over one hundred percent. Roughly, we might be able to conclude that, given that the adjustment for age has already occurred in the original numbers for pancreatic (women), the success of this particular model is high.

As usual, we jump now to the bottom box to check correlations mainly to make sure that the items used for explaining this pattern are not linked with each other. This is a requirement of the method even though, in reality, we must often settle for items that are connected to some extent. Looking at the two items here, state altitude [altstate] and drinking wine [ethpcwyn] [ethanol, (a scientific word for alcohol) per capita - wine], we are pleased to find that there is virtually no connection between them (corr. .001). The model is "clean".

Table 9-6 The Pancreatic cancer model (women): a connection with drinking wine.

Model Summary

Model	R	R Square	Adjusted R Square	Std. Error of the Estimate
1	.742[a]	.550	.532	.5302

a. Predictors: (Constant), ETHPCWYN, ALTSTATE

Coefficients[a]

Model		Unstandardized Coefficients		Standardized Coefficients	t	Sig.
		B	Std. Error	Beta		
1	(Constant)	8.856	.176		50.381	.000
	ALTSTATE	-2.465E-04	.000	-.584	-6.034	.000
	ETHPCWYN	2.297	.485	.458	4.738	.000

a. Dependent Variable: PANWIM60

Correlations

		ALTSTATE	ETHPCWYN	PANWIM60
ALTSTATE	Pearson Correlation	1	.001	-.583**
	Sig. (2-tailed)	.	.992	.000
	N	51	51	51
ETHPCWYN	Pearson Correlation	.001	1	.458**
	Sig. (2-tailed)	.992	.	.001
	N	51	51	51
PANWIM60	Pearson Correlation	-.583**	.458**	1
	Sig. (2-tailed)	.000	.001	.
	N	51	51	51

**. Correlation is significant at the 0.01 level (2-tailed).

In this case, both items are correlated with pancreatic cancer deaths. The correlation between pancreatic cancer and altitude is -.583**. This means that, as the elevation of a state goes higher, there are FEWER deaths from pancreatic cancer. Turned around, as the elevation gets lower with the lowest being around sea level, there are more deaths from pancreatic cancer. The correlation between wine drinking and pancreatic cancer deaths is +.458**. More wine drinking, more deaths from pancreatic cancer (among women).

The model itself is found in the middle box in Table 9-6. First, however, we will check statistical significance in the two columns to the right. Sig for both items is .000, excellent, and the t value is well above the required 2. For altitude it is 6 and for wine drinking it is well over 4. These results suggest the findings are solid.

As for the size of the connections with pancreatic cancer, we look to the Beta column now in the middle column of the second box down in Table 9-6. Ignoring the plus and minus signs (the plus only implied), the size of these numbers can be compared directly to each other to get a sense of the relative effect of each item on deaths from pancreatic cancer. Altitude is the larger connection (.584) and the connection with wine is slightly less (.458).

For the exact proportion, we add them both together (without the direction signs) and divide each by that number. 584+458=1036. 584/1036=.564. Altitude accounts for about 56 percent of the portion of the pattern between states that the model explains. 458/1036=.442. Drinking wine explains about 44 percent of the part of the explanation that the model explains.

More important, perhaps, is the part of the TOTAL explanation that these items account for. This is because the model as a whole succeeds in explaining the majority of the pattern (53.2 percent) which leaves a great deal unexplained. To find this, we convert the sum from the Beta column into the larger denominator that represent the total explanation, the part the model explains and the part it does not explain. 1036/.532=x/1. 1036=.532x. 1036/.532=x. x=1947.368. Now we divide each Beta value by this number to get the actual portion of the TOTAL explanation that each item represents. For altitude, this is 584/1947.368=.29989.

Altitude of the state represents 30 percent of the total explanation for the pattern between the states of pancreatic cancer among women. For wine, this is 458/1947.368=.2364. Wine drinking represents as an explanation of the total portion of the pattern between states in deaths from pancreatic cancer among women 23.6 percent. Drinking wine accounts for slightly less than a quarter of the total explanation of dying from pancreatic cancer among women as revealed in the pattern of deaths between states. Both numbers add together .29989+.2364=.536 which is a bit more than the actual Adjusted R Square of .532 but quite close.

As is our pattern, here we like to use the numbers in the B column of Table 9-6, which is an actual representation in equation form of the model explaining the original death rate numbers in Table 9-1. The middle number for altitude is simply another way of representing numbers small in size which translates to -.0002465. We like to use these numbers for constructing a best view of the death rate pattern often by zeroing out one of the items to see more clearly the effect of the other item, the one we find more interesting. In this case, however, the older age item is not there (as the numbers have already been adjusted for age to begin with).

Both items, however, are interesting and contribute substantially to the pattern. And yet, even though the connection with altitude is intriguing, more deaths the lower people live, my attention is naturally drawn to wine drinking. Perhaps the "best view" for me would be one where we zero out the effect for altitude to focus on the effect of wine drinking on dying from pancreatic cancer.

We can do this by using the average value for altitude, the mean of all the states, when we run the equation, while using the ACTUAL number for wine drinking in a state (found in Table 9-4). We do this in SPSS 11 from the data file by pulling down the "transform" menu and highlighting "compute". We can call the list panwine (for pancreatic wine). Using the numbers in the B column of the middle box of Table 9-6, we can now construct a list for this best view which will show us the effect of wine specifically. The mean for state altitude in feet is 1725.35. panwine = 8.856 - (.0002465 * 1725.35) + (2.297 * ethpcwyn).

Instructing the program to run the equation results in Table 9-7 panwine. "Best view" look at death rates from pancreatic cancer among women highlighting the effect of drinking wine (bad) while zeroing out the effect of living at lower elevation (bad).

Table 9-7 [panwine] pancreatic wine.

Best view look at death rate from pancreatic cancer among women by state highlighting the effect of drinking wine (more deaths) while largely zeroing out the effect of living at lower elevation (such as sea level)(more deaths).

State	Rate	State	Rate
West Virginia	8.64	Minnesota	9.05
Mississippi	8.64	Maryland	9.10
Utah	8.68	Montana	9.10
Oklahoma	8.71	Virginia	9.12
Arkansas	8.71	Maine	9.19
Iowa	8.71	Arizona	9.19
Kentucky	8.73	Illinois	9.23
South Dakota	8.73	Idaho	9.26
North Dakota	8.73	Alaska	9.26
Kansas	8.75	New York	9.30
Alabama	8.78	Hawaii	9.30
Tennessee	8.80	Florida	9.33
Wyoming	8.82	Colorado	9.33
Ohio	8.84	Washington	9.42
Nebraska	8.84	New Jersey	9.42
Indiana	8.87	Oregon	9.46
South Carolina	8.87	Rhode Island	9.49
Pennsylvania	8.89	Vermont	9.51
Texas	8.89	Delaware	9.51
Michigan	8.94	Connecticut	9.56
Missouri	8.94	California	9.58
Louisiana	8.96	Massachusetts	9.58
North Carolina	8.98	New Hampshire	9.69
New Mexico	8.98	Nevada	9.85
Georgia	9.00	District	10.25
Wisconsin	9.03		

In this pancreatic death rate list, West Virginia is the state with the lowest death rate of around 9 deaths per hundred thousand. District (of Columbia), Washington DC, is the "state" with the highest death rate of around 10 deaths. Compared with the lowest death rate state, the death rate in the highest state is as follows. 8.64/100=10.25/x. 1025=8.64x. 1025/8.64=x. x=118.63. The death rate in the highest state is 18.63 percent higher. Rounding, it is a bit less than a fifth higher. This is another way to understand that effect of wine drinking on death rates from pancreatic cancer.

Some thoughts now on what these results might tell us about pancreatic cancer itself. Of course, these thoughts are speculation. The link with elevation, the one that is less exciting but larger in size, is noteworthy because, in an alternative model not shown, there was a similar connection with lung cancer. There are fewer deaths from both cancers at higher elevation. These effects are in the same directions (confusing myself momentarily). For pancreatic cancer, lower elevation is linked with more deaths. For lung cancer (in this alternative model) lower elevation is also linked with more deaths. This could be the context for understanding the connection between pancreatic cancer and drinking wine.

First my sincere apologies for uncovering this unpleasant finding that drinking wine might be linked with pancreatic cancer, the ultimate "death sentence" cancer among the many kinds. Like my finding earlier about having a dog, I dislike having the role of telling people that an activity that they enjoy might have negative health consequences. Perhaps more than any other kind of alcohol, there is a well developed culture around wine drinking with a great deal to learn about it as it has become for many a full blown hobby. Wine loving Americans who redo their kitchens are sometimes installing a special wine refrigerator for keeping wine in the optimal conditions. This study suggests, however, that drinking wine might account for between less than a fifth and a quarter of the pattern across the country in how death rates vary by state from pancreatic cancer.

Why might this be? The two results taken together suggest (vaguely) to me that both involve some problem with breathing. Higher elevation speeds breathing making it more frequent. As the air is thinner, this allows for less airway resistance, particularly while sleeping during the night. Higher elevation is linked with fewer deaths from pancreatic cancer.

Conversely, wine, as one choice among several categories of alcoholic beverages, slows breathing. There might be other ways as well that drinking alcohol might affect breathing in a detrimental way. The impact could also be felt most importantly during sleep as typically, people drink alcohol at night during social situations. This slower breathing brought about by drinking wine might be a possible reason why wine is linked with more deaths from pancreatic cancer.

One final way to see the size of the effect of drinking wine on deaths from pancreatic cancer is by simply looking at the zero order correlation between the consumption of wine and pancreatic cancer. For this model, this simple view is appropriate given that both items in Table 9-6, the model, are so cleanly uncorrelated. That correlation (between drinking wine and pancreatic cancer) is +.458**.

At this eleventh hour, I did some preliminary checking for pancreatic deaths among men, and to my surprise, there is no reliable connection between death rates among men from pancreatic cancer and any measures for alcohol drinking including wine. As it stand now, it is important to note that this finding applies only for women. The correlation between death rates for women and for men from pancreatic cancer is only +.721**. This could either mean that the pattern for each gender is different or that there is a problem with the numbers for men.

Looking at the correlations between women death rates and the alternative alcohol measure of alcohol per capita (which drops out of the model), I see that it is unreliable at .329*. This allows me to strengthen the conclusion about pancreatic cancer and alcohol among women. It appears more clearly to me now that the connection is specifically with drinking wine and NOT with alcohol in general. From these further checks at "five minutes to midnight" before concluding the chapter, the association between alcohol and pancreatic cancer only applies to wine specifically.

What about men? To what extent does the finding linking wine with pancreatic cancer apply to men given that the starting set of numbers is deaths from pancreatic cancer among women? In even later thinking about this during the night, I have changed my opinion on this question.

Obviously, there is no specific evidence linking wine to dying from pancreatic cancer for men. I was ready to, thus, conclude, that the link applies only for women. Now, however, like my interpretation in other parts of this research, I believe the most successful model among several is, generally speaking, the most reliable for making deductions about the larger population of interest. In this case, we are speaking about such a population including men as well. The less successful set of numbers for men is most likely because there is "something wrong" with those numbers. As an example, some crass errors might have crept in while transposing, so easy to occur in this kind of work.

In short, I believe it might be best to ignore the work on the unsuccessful model for men and to, rather, focus on the successful model for women. Furthermore, I now believe, despite the conflicting results, that the model for women applies to men as well. This is my best guess. While lacking direct evidence that such is the case, the most reasonable conclusion is that the result linking wine drinking with pancreatic cancer applies not only for women but for men as well.

Chapter 10. Adult Leukemia Linked with Too Strong Earth Magnetism (from Living "North") and with Having a Dog

The estimated number of people who were expected to die from leukemia in 2015 is 24,450. In this chapter, we look at deaths from leukemia in the population that is age 18 and over and, thus, we look at adults only. In so doing, we exclude childhood leukemia. The age 18 and over cutoff is the case for all of the models in this research.

For the years 2011-2013, the death rate from leukemia (age 18+, crude) is 9.5 deaths per hundred thousand people. This is for the US as a whole. In this same set of years, the total death rate from cancer is 241.4 and the death rate from all causes is 1047.0. What are leukemia deaths as a percent of all deaths from cancer? 9.5/241.4=x/100. 241.4x=950. x=950/241.4. x=3.935. Leukemia is about 3.9 percent of all deaths from cancer or about 4 percent. What percent of total deaths are from leukemia? 9.5/1047.0=x/100. 1047x=950. x=950/1047. x=.907. As a percent of all deaths, deaths from leukemia are about .9 percent (nine tenth of one percent) or a little under one percent.

We can begin by looking at Table 10-1 Adult Leukemia. Death rates from leukemia in 2011-2013 by state. Of course, this is the number of deaths per hundred thousand people. It goes from a low of about 5 deaths in Alaska to a high of about 13 deaths in West Virginia. Compared to the lowest state, how much higher is the death rate in the highest state? 5.3/100=12.5/x. 5.3x=1250. x=1250/5.3. x=235.85. The death rate from leukemia is over two and a third times higher in the highest state compared with the lowest.

Before presenting the leukemia death rate model in Table 10-5, it is useful to become familiar with the items that are part of that model. The first is the percent seniors. More seniors, more deaths from leukemia. Seniors is shown in Table 10-2 Seniors. Percent age 65 and over by state (2006). Alaska has the fewest seniors as a percent of the population, around 7 percent. Florida has the highest amount, about 17 percent. As both are no-state-income-tax states, I presume the difference in winter weather helps to explain this.

Table 10-1 Adult Leukemia.
Death rates from leukemia in 2011-2013 by state.

State	Rate	State	Rate
Alaska	5.3	Illinois	9.9
District	6.4	Mississippi	9.9
Utah	6.5	Montana	9.9
Hawaii	7.4	Oregon	10.1
Georgia	7.5	Michigan	10.2
Colorado	7.5	Rhode Island	10.3
Texas	7.9	Tennessee	10.3
New Mexico	8.0	Connecticut	10.4
California	8.1	Kentucky	10.5
Nevada	8.2	Nebraska	10.6
Virginia	8.3	Missouri	10.6
Maryland	8.8	Minnesota	10.7
Washington	8.9	Indiana	10.7
Idaho	8.9	Ohio	10.8
North Dakota	9.0	Alabama	10.8
Vermont	9.1	Florida	10.9
North Carolina	9.1	Kansas	11.0
New York	9.2	Arkansas	11.0
Louisiana	9.2	Oklahoma	11.0
New Jersey	9.3	Wyoming	11.1
South Carolina	9.3	Maine	11.3
Delaware	9.5	Wisconsin	11.4
Arizona	9.5	Pennsylvania	11.5
Massachusetts	9.8	Iowa	11.6
New Hampshire	9.8	South Dakota	11.9

Table 10-2 Older age.
Percent seniors (Age 65 and Over) in a state (2006)

State	%	State	%
Alaska	6.8	Kentucky	12.8
Utah	8.8	New Jersey	12.9
Georgia	9.8	Kansas	12.9
Texas	9.9	Oregon	12.9
Colorado	10.0	Wisconsin	13.0
California	10.8	New York	13.1
Nevada	11.1	Oklahoma	13.2
Idaho	11.5	Nebraska	13.3
Washington	11.5	Massachusetts	13.3
Virginia	11.6	Vermont	13.3
Maryland	11.6	Missouri	13.3
Illinois	12.0	Connecticut	13.4
Minnesota	12.1	Delaware	13.4
Wyoming	12.2	Alabama	13.4
North Carolina	12.2	Ohio	13.4
Louisiana	12.2	Montana	13.8
District	12.3	Rhode Island	13.9
New Mexico	12.4	Arkansas	13.9
New Hampshire	12.4	Hawaii	14.0
Indiana	12.4	South Dakota	14.2
Mississippi	12.4	North Dakota	14.6
Michigan	12.5	Iowa	14.6
Tennessee	12.7	Maine	14.6
Arizona	12.8	Pennsylvania	15.2
South Carolina	12.8	West Virginia	15.3
		Florida	16.8

The next item that helps to explain the pattern of deaths from leukemia between all the states is geomagnetism, the size of the Earth's magnetic field on the ground. Generally speaking, it goes up the more north the state happens to be, the closer it happens to be situated to the magnetic pole which is not far from the regular geographic pole. As the magnetic field on the ground increases in size (as you drive north), the more deaths there are from leukemia.

The size of the magnetic field in the largest city of each state can be seen in Table 10-3 Geomagnetism [geomag15]. Size of Earth magnetism on the ground in nanoTeslas (nT) on September 3, 2015 using a NOAA online magnetic field calculator (entering latitude, longitude and altitude) for the largest city of the state. [My notes record the source as ngdc.noaa.gov/geomng-web/#1grfwmm gps.wmm(2014-2019). 2015 9.3. Other notes add the following: wmm (world magnetic model) elevation GPS feet. Lat N, Long W. 2015 9th month, 3rd day]. For reasons involving the importance of this finding for several cancer death rates, I took the time to update this item to add another test.

The geomagnetism low for major cities in each state is for Hawaii at about 35000 nanoTeslas. The highest magnetic field is in the state of North Dakota where it is about 56000 nanoTeslas. What is the comparison between the lowest and highest level? 34996.6/100=55897.9/x. 34996.6x=5589790. x=5589790/34996.6. x=159.7. Compared to the lowest geomagnetism level in Honolulu Hawaii, the level in Fargo North Dakota is close to 60 percent higher.

In a technical note for this item [geomag15], I did not use my OWN selection of cities which I chose by largest population size but rather the selection of the city made for the UV Index. Besides being updated for population changes in the intervening years, I wanted to have an exact match to make a good comparison between these two items which happen to be highly correlated with each other but in a negative direction (corr. geomagnetism in 2015 [geomag15] and UV index annual in 1996 [ultra96] = -.920**).

We can think about driving north from Key West Florida to Bar Harbor Maine or from San Diego California to Seattle Washington - having done both drives. The size of Earth magnetism goes up while the strength of the sun's ultraviolet component goes down. It so happens that Earth magnetism as well as insufficient ultraviolet (as you drive north) are both possible items which help explain the pattern of various kinds of cancer in the United States. For this reason, it was important to have the most valid comparison for testing both items to see which of them is the best fit for each different kind of cancer.

Table 10-3 [geomag15] geomagnetism in 2015.

Size of Earth magnetism on the ground in nanoTeslas (nT) in the largest city of the state. I use a USGS online magnetic field calculator on September 3, 2015 entering the city latitude, longitude and altitude.

State	nT	State	nT
Hawaii	34996.6	Rhode Island	51955.2
Florida	44113.5	Kentucky	52011.7
California	46944.4	Connecticut	52166.9
Louisiana	47430.1	Massachusetts	52190.6
Arizona	47717.9	Colorado	52238.1
Alabama	47803.6	Missouri	52475.3
South Carolina	48479.6	Maine	52655.8
Nevada	48755.1	New Hampshire	52657.3
Mississippi	48850.0	Idaho	52728.3
Texas	49072.0	Oregon	52752.7
Georgia	49357.7	Indiana	52820.1
New Mexico	49413.3	Wyoming	52971.5
North Carolina	50039.0	Ohio	53320.3
Virginia	50246.6	Vermont	53498.6
Tennessee	50447.8	Washington	53709.9
Oklahoma	50492.4	Nebraska	53711.6
Arkansas	50562.2	Michigan	53869.0
Delaware	51328.5	Iowa	53872.8
New Jersey	51350.9	Illinois	53946.9
District	51531.8	Wisconsin	54436.0
Maryland	51536.0	South Dakota	54745.2
Pennsylvania	51679.7	Montana	54820.5
West Virginia	51733.3	Minnesota	55352.8
Kansas	51756.4	Alaska	55654.9
Utah	51892.2	North Dakota	55897.9
New York	51922.3		

Table 10-4 dog.
Percent of households in a state with a dog (one or more).

State	%	State	%
District	6.9	Indiana	33.6
New York	21.9	Washington	34.0
Massachusetts	22.5	Alaska	34.0
Rhode Island	22.6	South Dakota	34.3
New Jersey	23.1	Arizona	34.4
Connecticut	25.2	Kansas	34.8
New Hampshire	25.5	Nebraska	35.2
Vermont	25.8	Kentucky	35.4
Maryland	26.6	Louisiana	35.7
Maine	26.9	South Carolina	35.8
North Dakota	27.6	Georgia	35.8
Pennsylvania	27.7	Alabama	35.9
Florida	28.2	Tennessee	36.0
Wisconsin	28.2	North Carolina	36.9
Illinois	28.3	Missouri	36.9
Minnesota	28.5	Mississippi	37.5
Michigan	30.2	Nevada	37.8
Ohio	30.4	Colorado	38.1
Delaware	31.2	West Virginia	39.3
Virginia	31.3	Idaho	39.4
Iowa	31.6	Montana	40.0
Utah	31.8	Texas	40.9
Hawaii	32.0	Arkansas	41.2
California	32.0	New Mexico	41.3
Oregon	32.9	Oklahoma	41.7
		Wyoming	47.9

The third and final item in the upcoming leukemia model is households with a dog. The higher the percent of households with a dog, the more deaths from leukemia in that state. The state with the fewest households with a dog (for its population size) is "District", Washington, District of Columbia, where about 7 percent of households have a dog, one or more. The highest percent is in Wyoming where about 48 percent of households have a dog. How many times higher is the highest state compared with the lowest? Perhaps we should skip over Washington DC whose low number of households with dogs surely says something about the distinctive demographic nature of the population in that area. We will use for this comparison the second lowest dog-household state, New York, where about 22 percent of households have a dog. 21.9/100=47.9/x. 4790=21.9x. x=4790/21.9. x=218.72. Compared with New York, over twice as many households have a dog in Wyoming.

Now we are ready to review the actual leukemia model in Table 10-5. As is our pattern, we start with the bottom box to look at correlations between the three items in the upcoming main model. It is important that they be as uncorrelated as possible for purposes of instilling confidence that the model will be valid. We start here because it is a requirement of the method itself.

This model is "clean" as all three items: age 65, geomagnetism and dog are not significantly correlated with each other (no stars). The resulting correlation numbers are low in size.

We can also glance at the bottom row at the zero order correlations with the item of interest: leukemia. Leukemia is highly correlated with older age (.750**). For the other two items, magnetism and having a dog, we have to wait for the full model to first "pull out" this large effect of age to bring into view the connection between these other items and leukemia.

About ready for the leukemia model now, we start in the top box in Table 10-5 to see that the Adjusted R Square is .752. The model as a whole, with its three items of age, magnetism and having a dog, explains over 75 percent of the pattern between states.

Finally reaching the actual model for leukemia death rates now in the middle box in Table 10-5, we start on the right with those two columns about statistical signficance. Sig. for all three is .000, very good. The t values are correspondingly high. While they need to be over 2, the t value for age is near 12, for magnetism over 5 and for dog over 4.

Table 10-5 The Adult Leukemia Model:

The role of higher Earth magnetism (more north, more deaths) and having a dog (more deaths)

Model Summary

Model	R	R Square	Adjusted R Square	Std. Error of the Estimate
1	.876[a]	.767	.752	.7520

a. Predictors: (Constant), DOGHOUSE, GEOMAG15, AGE65IN6

	Model	Unstandardized Coefficients		Standardized Coefficients	t	Sig.
		B	Std. Error	Beta		
1	(Constant)	-10.909	2.111		-5.167	.000
	AGE65IN6	.767	.065	.849	11.767	.000
	GEOMAG15	1.649E-04	.000	.367	5.126	.000
	DOGHOUSE	7.332E-02	.016	.330	4.568	.000

a. Dependent Variable: LEUK1113

		AGE65IN6	GEOMAG15	DOGHOUSE	LEUK1113
AGE65IN6	Pearson Correlation	1	-.114	-.175	.750**
	Sig. (2-tailed)	.	.426	.220	.000
	N	51	51	51	51
GEOMAG15	Pearson Correlation	-.114	1	-.114	.232
	Sig. (2-tailed)	.426	.	.425	.101
	N	51	51	51	51
DOGHOUSE	Pearson Correlation	-.175	-.114	1	.139
	Sig. (2-tailed)	.220	.425	.	.329
	N	51	51	51	51
LEUK1113	Pearson Correlation	.750**	.232	.139	1
	Sig. (2-tailed)	.000	.101	.329	.
	N	51	51	51	51

**. Correlation is significant at the 0.01 level (2-tailed).

Next is the Beta column in the middle which gives us an idea of the relative size of each of the three items compared to the other two. Of course, the items are in size order with the effect of older age on the pattern being the biggest in size.

These size comparisons can be easily quantified relative to each other. Then, they can be seen as a portion of the entire size that the item has on the pattern across the states. This includes the part of the explanation that the model explains and the part that it does not.

For the relative size of each item, we add up the three numbers in the Beta column in Table 10-5. For this, I ignore decimals as well as signs (+ or -). 849+367+330=1546. What is the size of the age effect? 849/1546=54.9. Speaking of the portion of the explanation (of the pattern between states) that the models succeeds in capturing (the 75.2 percent), older age explains 54.9, or about 55 percent. How much does Earth magnetism explain? 367/1546=.237. Of this portion of the explanation that the model captures, Earth magnetism explains about 24 percent of it.

Lastly is having a dog. 330/1546=.213. Of this portion of the pattern in leukemia death rate variations between states, households with dogs explains 21 percent or a bit over a fifth of the pattern.

More interesting, perhaps, is the role of each item as part of the total explanation of the pattern, the part captured by the model and the part not. From the Adjusted R Square of .752, we know that, while the model explains some 75 percent of the pattern, there is another quarter that has eluded our best efforts. How much does each item succeed in accounting for as a portion of the total 100 percent of the pattern? .752/1546=1/x. .752x=1546. x=1546/.752. x=2055.85. This is our new denominator. We can now divide each Beta by this larger denominator to get the portion of the total explanation for each item.

Age is first. 849/2055.85=.413. Older age accounts for 41.3 percent of the total pattern of difference in leukemia death rates between states. Next is geomagnetism. 367/2055.85=.1785. Of the total pattern, geomagnetism accounts for about 17.9 percent. Lastly is having a dog. 330/2055.85=.161. Households with dogs accounts for 16.1 percent of the total pattern in leukemia deaths between states.

Finally we can move to the B column in the middle box to have our first look at the actual equation. These numbers represent, in equation form, the model result. It is an attempt to account for the pattern of differences in leukemia death rates in Table 10-1 Adult Leukemia. The unfamiliar form of the numbers for magnetism and dog simply represent a different way of saying we need to move the decimal to the left by four places for magnetism and by two places for dog.

We can now use this equation to come up with a "best view" look at the pattern of leukemia deaths between states. Once again for this cancer, older age is less interesting because it seems to be common that the more people in a state who are in this older age category, the more people who die from cancer. Such is also the case typically for dying in general but each death category has to be examined to be sure. For this cancer, the numbers suggest that older age is such a big part of the story that it simply must be part of the model (as a control) before we can have a valid look at the other items that might be involved.

Not only is age less interesting to us but the other two items are both interesting. While always a judgment call at this point, I imagine that the best view would include the effect of both of these: magnetism as well as having a dog.

A plan of action has now been finalized. Using the original equation, we, of course, DO capture the effect of age in a general way but to "zero out the effect of older age, we use the mean (average) value for age which happens to be 12.653. (The average percent seniors in a state in the United States is a little under 13 percent of the population). For the other two items, as we ARE interested in the effect of these, we plug in the ACTUAL values for each state. We find this for magnetism in Table 10-3 and for households with a dog in Table 10-4. Now we are ready to build the equation which will produce our "best view" custom look at the pattern of leukemia deaths across the United States.

We use the numbers in the B column combining them with either the mean value or the actual value. We instruct the computer program to do this. From the data file in SPSS 11, we pull down "transform", highlight "compute" and we will call this "best view" list Leukmagd (leukemia magnetism dog). Leukmagd= -10.909 + (.767 * 12.653) + (.0001649 * geomag15) + (.07332 * doghouse).

In Table 10-6, we can see the result of running the equation. Table 10-6 leukmagd (leukemia magnetism dog). "Best view" look at death rates from leukemia by state after accounting for the connection with older age (bad, more deaths) in order to see more clearly the effect of Earth magnetism (bad) and households with a dog (bad).

Table 10-6 [leukmagd] leukemia magnetism dog. Best view look at death rate from leukemia by state between 2011 and 2013 after accounting for the effect of older age (more deaths). This allows us to see the effects more clearly of both Earth magnetism (more deaths) as well as having a dog (more deaths).

State	Rate	State	Rate
Hawaii	6.91	Tennessee	9.75
District	7.80	Illinois	9.77
Florida	8.14	Ohio	9.82
California	8.88	Wisconsin	9.84
New Jersey	8.96	Kansas	9.88
New York	8.96	Texas	9.89
Rhode Island	9.02	Michigan	9.89
Massachusetts	9.05	Oregon	9.91
Arizona	9.19	Kentucky	9.97
Louisiana	9.23	Indiana	9.97
Maryland	9.24	New Mexico	9.97
Connecticut	9.25	Iowa	10.00
Alabama	9.31	Minnesota	10.01
New Hampshire	9.35	North Dakota	10.04
Pennsylvania	9.35	Washington	10.15
Virginia	9.38	Arkansas	10.15
South Carolina	9.41	Missouri	10.15
Maine	9.45	Oklahoma	10.18
Vermont	9.51	Colorado	10.20
Delaware	9.55	West Virginia	10.21
Georgia	9.56	Nebraska	10.23
Mississippi	9.60	South Dakota	10.34
Nevada	9.61	Idaho	10.38
Utah	9.68	Alaska	10.47
North Carolina	9.75	Montana	10.77
		Wyoming	11.04

Unlike many other cancers, the ordering of this state list does not exactly correspond to any other list. It is different than the original state list of leukemia deaths in Table 10-1, of course, because we largely removed the effect of older age. It is also different, however, from the listing of states in Table 10-3 Geomagnetism. This is the case because, not only does geomagnetism vary here but so does having a dog in Table 10-4, both effects divided up in the equation based on their relative impact on leukemia (magnetism being the larger of the two).

Looking first at Table 10-6 leukmagd compared roughly with the original list in Table 10-1 for Adult Leukemia, it is obvious that these are different from each other. In the original list (Table 10-1), Alaska is the lowest leukemia deaths state but, in our best view list (Table 10-6), it moves down to almost the highest (third highest). This is largely due to the effect of older age because there are so few seniors in Alaska (as a percent of the population). We can see this in Table 10-2 Seniors.

"Seniors" is not the full explanation, however. Being so north on the map, Alaska has high geomagnetism (Table 10-3 Geomagnetism, showing Alaska as second highest). Of course, Alaska would be high then because more geomagnetism, more deaths from leukemia. As for households with a dog, Alaska is 28 lowest, close to the middle value of around number 26 (out of 51). Clearly, then, the main reason why Alaska has such a high predicted death rate from leukemia in this list in Table 10-6 is its high value for Earth magnetism on the ground (largely as a result of the extreme northern location of Anchorage Alaska).

In one more example for an individual state, we can look at Florida, quite high in the original leukemia death rate list in Table 10-1. In Table 10-6, this "best view" list shows Florida as third best, with among the fewest deaths from leukemia. Obviously, this is due to largely removing the effect of older age. Table 10-2 shows us that Florida has the highest percent of seniors as a part of the population.

Once again, while "Seniors" is a large part of the story explaining the change with the original list (Table 10-1), it is only part of the explanation. Starting with the smaller item, having a dog (Table 10-4), Florida is among the states with the fewest households with dogs, 13 lowest (out of 51). As having a dog is linked with deaths from leukemia, this would surely be part of the explanation for why Florida does so much "better" (with fewer deaths).

An even larger explanation is Earth magnetism. Because Florida is situated so far south, the level of geomagnetism is low. We see this in Table 10-3 showing that the size of geomagnetism in Florida is second lowest, with Hawaii the only state that is lower, largely reflecting Hawaii's much more southern location. This must also be a large part of the explanation.

For the state of Florida, after accounting for older age, this popular retirement state looks much better, a view that improves further by the relatively low number of households that have a dog (for the size of the population). The larger effect, however, is the low Earth magnetism for Miami Florida due to its southern location.

After a reconsideration with momentary misgivings, I now confirm a second time that the analysis presented here is correct. It represents the most fruitful choice for constructing a list of predicted death rates for this disease. While adjusting for older age in Table 10-6 is surely a big factor, I believe it is legitimate to point out the effect of the other two items as well when explaining the difference between our best view look in Table 10-6 with the original list in Table 10-1.

All three items in the model help to explain the dramatic difference in the ordering of the states and the predicted death rates which result (in Table 10-6). As far as the work here goes, given that we only explain three quarters of the pattern, the list of states in Table 10-6 is indeed, the "best view", in my judgment.

As an aside, some readers might disagree with my decision for constructing the best view, unhappy that I included having a dog. A dog, they might say, is a matter of choice, perhaps more the case for those who do not now have one or who never had one. They might want to have a best view constructed only from those features that are intrinsic to the particular state such as the magnetism on the ground in that location.

I wish to point out that this listing of states can already be found in Table 10-3 Geomagnetism. While that table does not provide a predicted death rate from leukemia, the order of such a list would be identical to that table because, in that alternative "best view" decision, it is only geomagnetism that would be allowed to vary.

I will conclude with thoughts about the results and how they might help to illuminate the nature of leukemia. I fear I have little profound to say and hope that others might be able to use these connections with greater insight into the nature of this cancer.

Beginning with older age, the connection with more deaths in a state is solid and large in size. The connection between older age and cancer is very important. For these models, it is essential to include "age" as a "control" before proceeding further. This is largely the case because of its big size. Older people are more likely to die from leukemia and the same is true for cancer in general. The same is also true for death from all causes (taken together).

Perhaps cellular senescence is involved, with shortening telomeres. This could be one reason for unrestrained cell growth. I suspect that it is the cell killing mechanism that fails to do its job leading to an overabundance of defective cells.

This leaves two additional connections uncovered in this research and I will start with dog. More households in a state which have a dog, more deaths from leukemia in that state. What might this connection mean? I am not sure. Perhaps dogs get cancer and somehow give it to the humans with whom they are in contact? Might the dander from a dog get into the lungs of people suggesting a reduction in breathing efficiency?

Most interesting of these three items is the connection between higher Earth magnetism on the ground and dying from leukemia (on a state level). While I am not certain, it is not likely that this would implicate magnetic fields whose origin is people-manipulated. Earth magnetism is, in effect, DC, Direct Current, whereas people-harnessed electricity gives off fields that are AC fields, from Alternating Current. Strangely, for this very cancer among children, the matter of nearness to power lines (whose moving electricity gives off magnetic fields) has been examined with results that are generally unimpressive.

The other difference is the size of Earth magnetism being so much smaller. Apparently, however, these differences in the Earth's magnetic field (which vary in size by about 60 percent) might constitute sufficient variation to be linked with dying from leukemia. This is despite the small absolute size of Earth magnetism on the ground. As best as we know, humankind developed right here on this planet so it does not seem that unreasonable to suggest the possibility that this geological attribute of magnetism might be responsible for an effect on human health.

While I believe the result to be valid as stated, higher geomagnetism, more deaths from leukemia, I tend to think this link might help us to uncover OTHER things possessing magnetism, perhaps from the ground, that would also be DC (Direct Current) in nature.

In concluding chapters, I suggest that this finding linking greater Earth magnetism with more deaths from leukemia might actually be misspecified. There, I present additional evidence which points to this alternative possibility.

Chapter 11. Prostate Cancer Linked with Living "North" Due to the Earth's Stronger Magnetic Field

We begin the research on dying from prostate cancer with the actual death rates by state for men who died of prostate cancer in 2010, 2011, and 2012. The list of death rates by state can be found in Table 11-1.

As best as I can figure out, this is the death rate from prostate cancer per hundred thousand people and, therefore, it includes women even though only men have prostates. The actual rate among men only dying from this disease is about double in size. Leaving the numbers in terms of the diseases from which all people die is more useful for comparison with other cancers and other causes of death. In a general way, I sense it is also more valid to use this common way of representing the numbers for purposes of modeling.

Before deciding on numbers to use for a final model, I calculated that about 2.2 percent of men die from prostate cancer based on deaths between 2011 and 2013. (For those years, the death rate from all causes for men is 1076.1 and for prostate cancer 23.7. 23.7/1076.1=.022 or 2.2 percent).

As usual, we use the numbers in Table 11-1 as the starting place and aim to build a model which explains the pattern of differences from state to state revealed in these numbers.

Looking over Table 11-1, we see that the lowest death rate from prostate cancer is in Alaska where about 7 men (people) die per hundred thousand population. The highest number of deaths per hundred thousand is in "District" (Washington DC) where about 15 men die.

Now we can become familiar with the items in the final model before turning to the model itself. In a rare decision, I do want to mention a "null" finding, that there is no connection between percent African American and dying from prostate cancer. It fails the stringent statistical test at the .01 level used in all of these models.

I will once again confirm this null finding for the final model. Using the model in Table 11-4, the middle and top boxes, adding percent African American has a Sig. value of .061, not significant (even at the .05 level). This means that the model fails to show a connection between percent black and men dying from prostate cancer to a solid enough degree that it can be discerned statistically.

Table 11-1 [pros1012] Death rate from prostate cancer in 2010-2012 per hundred thousand people (including women).

State	Rate	State	Rate
Alaska	7.3	Louisiana	12.1
Texas	8.8	West Virginia	12.1
Hawaii	9.4	New Mexico	12.5
Georgia	10.4	Oklahoma	12.5
Utah	10.7	Delaware	12.6
Colorado	10.7	Minnesota	12.6
California	10.7	Rhode Island	12.7
Nevada	10.8	Ohio	12.7
Virginia	10.9	Maine	13.0
Kentucky	10.9	Nebraska	13.2
Maryland	11.0	South Carolina	13.2
Mississippi	11.1	Arkansas	13.3
Wyoming	11.4	Pennsylvania	13.5
New York	11.5	Iowa	13.6
Washington	11.6	Idaho	13.7
New Jersey	11.7	North Dakota	13.8
Kansas	11.7	Wisconsin	13.8
Illinois	11.7	Oregon	13.8
Massachusetts	11.7	Florida	13.8
Arizona	11.8	South Dakota	14.1
Tennessee	11.8	Alabama	14.1
North Carolina	11.9	Vermont	14.1
New Hampshire	12.0	Montana	14.7
Connecticut	12.0	Missouri	14.8
Indiana	12.1	District	14.8
Michigan	12.1		

Moving to the two items that did make it into the final model, the first is our familiar older "age", the percent of the population that is in the senior category of age 65 and over. The more such older people, the more deaths from prostate cancer. Prostate cancer is thus, related, not surprisingly, to being "older".

This list for percent age 65 can be found in Table 11-2. The second lowest state in terms of its population of seniors as a percent is Utah with about 9 percent seniors. The third highest percent is in Pennsylvania with around 15 percent seniors.

The second item, of two in the prostate model, is one of my early lists for geomagnetism, from the USGS in about early 1998. I seem to recall receiving a floppy disc with a geomagnetism calculator based on the latest model-based values. I plugged in coordinates for my 51 cities for latitude, longitude and altitude (as best as I recall). This gave me values in nanoTeslas (nT) for each city. Each number is the geomagnetism calculator answer for the size of the strength of geomagnetism on the ground in that location. These values for geomagnetism appear in Table 11-3 [magnetic].

While I also have other calculations using a more recent calculator available online, this is the item that worked best, linked most clearly and strongly with deaths from prostate cancer by state during the period 2010-2012. Therefore, it is this version of geomagnetism that I selected for the final prostate model.

These numbers vary rather roughly with latitude with the lowest values closer to the equator and the highest values closest to the pole, actually the geomagnetic pole rather than the geographic one.

Not surprisingly, in the US, the lowest value for geomagnetism on the ground is in Hawaii, so far south and quite close to the equator with a value of about 36000 nanoTeslas. The highest value is for North Dakota at around 58000 nanoTeslas. Surprisingly, Alaska, even though it is so much farther north, is some 13 states away from the highest value perhaps because North Dakota is actually closer to the location of the nearest geomagnetic pole.

The higher the strength of predicted geomagnetism in the largest city of the state, the more deaths there are from prostate cancer in that state.

Table 11-2 Older Age.
Percent Age 65 and Over in each state (2006)

State	%	State	%
		Kentucky	12.8
Alaska	6.8	New Jersey	12.9
Utah	8.8	Kansas	12.9
Georgia	9.8	Oregon	12.9
Texas	9.9	Wisconsin	13.0
Colorado	10.0	New York	13.1
California	10.8	Oklahoma	13.2
Nevada	11.1	Nebraska	13.3
Idaho	11.5	Massachusetts	13.3
Washington	11.5	Vermont	13.3
Virginia	11.6	Missouri	13.3
Maryland	11.6	Connecticut	13.4
Illinois	12.0	Delaware	13.4
Minnesota	12.1	Alabama	13.4
Wyoming	12.2	Ohio	13.4
North Carolina	12.2	Montana	13.8
Louisiana	12.2	Rhode Island	13.9
District	12.3	Arkansas	13.9
New Mexico	12.4	Hawaii	14.0
New Hampshire	12.4	South Dakota	14.2
Indiana	12.4	North Dakota	14.6
Mississippi	12.4	Iowa	14.6
Michigan	12.5	Maine	14.6
Tennessee	12.7	Pennsylvania	15.2
Arizona	12.8	West Virginia	15.3
South Carolina	12.8	Florida	16.8

Table 11-3 [magnetic] geomagnetism.
Earth magnetism on the ground in the largest city of the state (by population) in nanoTeslas. For this version, I used a USGS calculator back in the late 1990s.

State	nT	State	nT
Hawaii	35625.4	Rhode Island	54405.8
Florida	46661.5	Oregon	54488.2
California	48806.5	Colorado	54495.4
Texas	49535.4	Massachusetts	54569.3
Arizona	49659.1	Kentucky	54602.1
Louisiana	49840.3	Connecticut	54625.9
Alabama	50301.8	Idaho	54747.8
Nevada	50726.3	Missouri	54943.7
South Carolina	51040.2	Maine	54957.6
Mississippi	51318.5	New Hampshire	55023.4
New Mexico	51567.1	Wyoming	55245.4
Georgia	52012.6	Alaska	55332.5
North Carolina	52601.4	Indiana	55391.8
Arkansas	52766.1	Washington	55578.2
Virginia	52847.1	Ohio	55844.2
Oklahoma	52918.3	Vermont	55849.6
Tennessee	53024.6	Nebraska	56143.5
New Jersey	53819.1	Michigan	56346.6
Utah	53981.5	Iowa	56382.3
District	54012.4	Illinois	56456.8
Maryland	54145.9	Wisconsin	56977.3
Delaware	54195.8	Montana	57023.5
Kansas	54198.2	South Dakota	57158.0
Pennsylvania	54228.3	Minnesota	57859.2
West Virginia	54322.4	North Dakota	58249.5
New York	54404.6		

Table 11-4 The Prostate Cancer Model: A connection with higher Earth magnetism in more northern locations (more deaths)

Model Summary

Model	R	R Square	Adjusted R Square	Std. Error of the Estimate
1	.774[a]	.600	.583	.9837

a. Predictors: (Constant), MAGNETIC, AGE65IN6

Coefficients[a]

Model		Unstandardized Coefficients		Standardized Coefficients	t	Sig.
		B	Std. Error	Beta		
1	(Constant)	-4.392	2.389		-1.839	.072
	AGE65IN6	.627	.083	.688	7.530	.000
	MAGNETIC	1.620E-04	.000	.376	4.113	.000

a. Dependent Variable: PROS1012

Correlations

		AGE65IN6	MAGNETIC	PROS1012
AGE65IN6	Pearson Correlation	1	-.029	.677**
	Sig. (2-tailed)	.	.839	.000
	N	51	51	51
MAGNETIC	Pearson Correlation	-.029	1	.356*
	Sig. (2-tailed)	.839	.	.010
	N	51	51	51
PROS1012	Pearson Correlation	.677**	.356*	1
	Sig. (2-tailed)	.000	.010	.
	N	51	51	51

**. Correlation is significant at the 0.01 level (2-tailed).
*. Correlation is significant at the 0.05 level (2-tailed).

Having introduced the items in the final model, we can now turn to the prostate model in Table 11-4. We begin, as usual, with the bottom box of correlations to ensure the level of connectedness between the two items is low. This fulfills the requirement of the method and helps to ensure that our results are not misleading at least based on one common cause of error. Older age and Earth magnetism are basically uncorrelated (-.029), tiny, with no stars meaning no statistically significant connection between them.

We now glance at the bottom row showing the zero order correlation between the matter of interest here, deaths from prostate cancer, and each item. First, we see that there is a strong connection between older age and prostate cancer of (+).677** (more older people, more deaths). The connection between Earth magnetism and prostate cancer, however, is modest both in size and solidness (+).256* (only one star).

Apparently, for this connection between geomagnetism and prostate cancer to become evident, we must first separate the large effect of older age. This happens next in the two item final model. This model is a view of the independent effect of each item on prostate cancer after already accounting for the other. This is when we should see the main connection here between Earth magnetism and dying from prostate cancer.

Next we look at the top box in Table 11-4 to see the Adjusted R Square for the entire model of .583. This means that the model explains 58.3 percent of the pattern of difference between states in the original list of prostate cancer deaths in Table 11-1. Relative to the models here, this is somewhat on the low side due to an unexplained difficulty in doing the model for this cancer, getting the numbers to "sing". On the positive side, however, the final model is "solid" as we shall see next.

Moving now to the most important middle box in Table 11-4, we can now begin to evaluate the final model. As usual, we begin with the test of statistical significance in the first two columns on the right. Starting on the extreme right we see the Sig. column. Both items of older age and Earth magnetism are linked with prostate cancer "solidly" with Sig. values of .000, the best. These numbers are based on the "t" values in the next column which need to be above 2. They are both well above. For age, the t value is almost 8, very high, and for Earth magnetism, the t value is about 4, also good.

Next we can begin to evaluate the question of the size of these connections with prostate cancer in the Beta column. Of course, both connections with prostate cancer are "positive" in direction. The implied plus sign means more seniors, more prostate cancer deaths. More Earth magnetism, that is, stronger (roughly, more north), more deaths from prostate cancer. As for size, the effect of age is much larger.

We can use these numbers to get a clearer view of size first treating what we found as 100 percent. Second, we will use the same numbers to figure out the broader question of how much of the possible total explanation each finding represents.

Starting with the first matter now, we add both numbers together without the decimals and the signs (an implied plus sign). 688+376=1064. For older age, 688/1064=.6466. Of the portion of the explanation we succeeded in discovering, older age represents 64.7 percent of the total. For Earth magnetism, 376/1064=.353. Earth magnetism represents 35.3 percent of the part of the explanation that we found, a little over a third.

Now, as a portion of the total possible explanation, we need to change the denominator using the old one of 1064, knowing that this represents 58.3 percent of the total explanation (from the Adjusted R Square in the top box of Table 11-4). 1064/58.3=x/100. 58.3x=106400. x=106400/58.3. x=1825.04, the new denominator.

For older age, we can find how much it represents as a portion of the total possible explanation by doing the following. 688/1825.04=.377 or 37.7 percent. Earth magnetism represents 376/1825.04=.206 or 20.6 percent of the total explanation.

So for this major finding linking the strength of Earth magnetism on the ground to dying from prostate cancer, we now know that it represents a bit over one fifth of the total explanation. We also know that the less exciting result linking prostate cancer deaths to older age, needed in the model as a "control", represents a bit over a third of the possible explanation.

Perhaps I can comment on the results thus far. As for the connection with older age, prostate cancer is solidly and sizably connected with older age. This is interesting to some extent as it is not always the case for every cancer and every disease even though, broadly speaking, it seems usually to be the case.

As for a connection between the size of Earth magnetism and dying from prostate cancer, readers will typically presume this is a case of misspecification - a connection with another item which also varies from south to north with geomagnetism. How could it be the size of the Earth's magnetic field itself given its small relative size, its weakness? The best defense of the finding is that, despite several attempts to test other such items, it is this - the size of Earth magnetism - that comes out as most clearly and strongly linked with dying from prostate cancer.

If it were the case, as I modestly argue here, that a too-strong magnetic field on the ground is involved with the rise of the prostate cancer death rate, I do not know what the mechanism would be. Nevertheless, the finding here, similar to the result with several other cancers, does suggest it as a possibility given the statistical evidence.

Now we can return to the B column in the middle box of Table 11-4 to use the actual equation to construct a clearer picture, a best view. The goal of this new picture of the pattern of deaths from prostate cancer is to create a version that provides greater insight when compared with the original list in Table 11-1. The best option for doing this seems obvious. We should minimize the effect of older age by allowing us to more clearly view the role of Earth magnetism as an explanation for deaths from prostate cancer.

We do this by using the average value for older age across all the states which happens to be 12.653, about 13 percent of the population. So for age, we use this value in the equation. For the item that truly interests us, however, Earth magnetism, we use the specific value for ground level Earth magnetism for each state from Table 11-3. That should result in what I call here the "best view" of death rates from prostate cancer.

We can do this now using the numbers from the B column from the middle box in Table 11-4. For magnetism, we will convert that number to a more familiar form by moving the decimal four places to the left. We will let the statistical software program run the equation (SPSS 11: from data file, "transform", "compute"). The equation is as follows: $-4.392 + (.627 * 12.653) + (.0001620 * magnetic)$. I will rerun it now as a check. Yes, it came out the same.

What results is a new look at prostate cancer death rates in Table 11-5, the look after having reduced the effect of older age by "holding it constant". Because only one item is allowed to vary in Table 11-5, the ordering of states is the same as the one in Table 11-3 Earth magnetism. What is new in this list is a predicted value for deaths per hundred thousand from prostate cancer.

In another attempt at clarity, this new list is a transposed version of the original numbers in Table 11-1 allowing us to see the effect of geomagnetism more clearly. Of course, this predicted estimate of death rates from prostate cancer is based on actual deaths in 2010-2012.

In Table 11-5, this new list shows the lowest prostate cancer death rate in Hawaii, the most southern state, with about 9 deaths. The highest predicted rate is in North Dakota, a northern part of the country, with about 13 deaths.

We can use this list to recheck the size of the magnetism effect. If the lowest death rate of 9.31 deaths is 100 percent, then 12.98 represents 100 plus how much? $9.31/100=12.98/x$. $9.31x=1298$. $x=1298/9.31$. $x=139.4$. Based on this result, then, prostate cancer death rates go up due to Earth magnetism by 39.4 percent.

For reasons unclear to me, this gives an impression of a larger role for Earth magnetism in the variation of death rates from prostate cancer. This compares to the "portion of the total explanation" evaluation (using the Beta numbers) which yielded a conclusion that geomagnetism was responsible for a bit over 20 percent of the total explanation for the difference between states in dying from prostate cancer. I guess these two "looks" at the matter of the role of Earth magnetism are not identical and need not be the same.

This new view from Table 11-5, based on not just the Beta numbers but rather the full equation (after controlling for age), appears to suggest that the role of geomagnetism as a factor affecting the number of deaths from prostate cancer is even more substantial in size.

In concluding chapters, I offer another interpretation for this "northern" pattern of prostate cancer deaths. There I suggest that there is evidence to suspect that this pattern is due not to Earth magnetism itself but rather to something else highly correlated with it – a different environmental factor.

Table 11-5 [prosmag1]

Best view predicted death rates from prostate cancer after controlling for older age (more deaths) while allowing to vary [magnetic] the strength of geomagnetism on the ground (more deaths).

Hawaii	9.31	Rhode Island	12.36
Florida	11.10	Oregon	12.37
California	11.45	Colorado	12.37
Texas	11.57	Massachusetts	12.38
Arizona	11.59	Kentucky	12.39
Louisiana	11.62	Connecticut	12.39
Alabama	11.69	Idaho	12.41
Nevada	11.76	Missouri	12.44
South Carolina	11.81	Maine	12.44
Mississippi	11.86	New Hampshire	12.46
New Mexico	11.90	Wyoming	12.49
Georgia	11.97	Alaska	12.51
North Carolina	12.06	Indiana	12.51
Arkansas	12.09	Washington	12.55
Virginia	12.10	Ohio	12.59
Oklahoma	12.11	Vermont	12.59
Tennessee	12.13	Nebraska	12.64
New Jersey	12.26	Michigan	12.67
Utah	12.29	Iowa	12.68
District	12.29	Illinois	12.69
Maryland	12.31	Wisconsin	12.77
Delaware	12.32	Montana	12.78
Kansas	12.32	South Dakota	12.80
Pennsylvania	12.33	Minnesota	12.91
West Virginia	12.34	North Dakota	12.98
New York	12.35		

Chapter 12. Ovarian Cancer and a Link with Not Strong Enough Sun

We begin with the list of ovarian cancer death rates by state in Table 12-1. This is for the years 2004, 2005 and 2006, a composite yearly average for each state. As I note on the table, the value for Alaska was missing, probably a mistake from copying my own data file and the actual number was no longer easily available. I used an overlapping set of years for that value from 2003-2005 as a replacement.

I had several such ovarian cancer death rate lists from recent years. I decide which to use usually from the general success of the model as revealed in the Adjusted R Square. For unknown reasons, this set of years worked far better than more recent ones.

I use the more common death rate based on the entire population including woman and men even though it is obvious that only woman die of it. At the risk of sounding silly, this is because men do not have certain body parts and, therefore, cannot die when these female parts become cancerous. This is also the case for uterine cancer deaths, as well as for cervical cancer deaths. Breast cancer is slightly different because men also have breasts and do also die from breast cancer even though, as a percent of all breast cancer deaths, the male component is very small (about one percent).

Speaking of ovarian and other specifically female cancers, the trans-gender issue complicates things somewhat. I presume that these internal female organs are not constructed for males who become transgender females. Obviously, for breasts, transgender females' breasts become enlarged but, in this case, given that men have breasts to start with, breast cancer is possible in both genders.

The death rate is given per hundred thousand population including men (who cannot get ovarian cancer). I tried using the rate among women only but returned to this more general format because the models appeared to work more successfully. The format as presented allows us to compare this cancer with others but we must remember that, among women only, the rate is about double (as best as I can figure out. I admit that I am very uncertain about this).

Looking more closely at the list for ovarian cancer death rates by state in Table 12-1, we see that the range goes from the lowest rate in Utah of about 5 (4.9) deaths per hundred thousand population (including men) to the highest of the 51 "states" which is Pennsylvania at about 10 (9.9) deaths per hundred thousand.

Table 12-1 [ovar46ak] ovarian 2004-2006 Alaska. Ovarian Cancer death rate by state between 2004 and 2006*, average annual, per hundred thousand population (including both genders). *Alaska from 2003-2005.

State	Rate	State	Rate
Utah	4.9	Missouri	7.8
Texas	5.6	Florida	7.9
Nevada	5.7	Alabama	7.9
Colorado	5.9	Michigan	7.9
Georgia	6.0	Tennessee	8.0
Hawaii	6.2	Maine	8.0
California	6.3	Indiana	8.0
Idaho	6.3	Ohio	8.0
Wyoming	6.3	Vermont	8.0
Arizona	6.5	South Dakota	8.0
New Mexico	6.5	Delaware	8.2
Louisiana	6.6	Nebraska	8.2
Mississippi	6.8	Connecticut	8.3
Arkansas	6.9	Wisconsin	8.3
Kentucky	7.0	New Jersey	8.4
South Carolina	7.2	Oregon	8.4
New Hampshire	7.2	New York	8.5
North Carolina	7.3	Massachusetts	8.6
Virginia	7.3	Montana	8.8
Maryland	7.3	West Virginia	8.9
Illinois	7.5	Iowa	9.1
Minnesota	7.5	North Dakota	9.1
Oklahoma	7.6	District	9.2
Kansas	7.7	Rhode Island	9.3
Alaska	7.7	Pennsylvania	9.9
Washington	7.7		

California is low (6.3), Florida is in the middle and New York is high, 9th highest of 51 (8.5) with my own state of Rhode Island second worst (9.3).

This is a short model that produces a rather high portion of the explained pattern between states (Adjusted R Square). The two items linked with ovarian cancer deaths in the model are older age and ultraviolet radiation. The higher the percent of older residents in the state, (age 65 and over), the higher the death rate from ovarian cancer. This is not a surprise.

The second connection is more interesting - ultraviolet. The stronger the ultraviolet is that reaches the ground over the course of the year, the LOWER the death rate from ovarian cancer. Another way of saying the same thing is this: the weaker the ultraviolet in sunlight reaching the ground in that location, the higher the death rate from ovarian cancer.

As has been the pattern in previous chapters, I make available the actual lists for each item in Tables 12-2 and 12-3. Table 12-2 is the Percent age 65 and Over in a state in 2006. Percent Seniors, a common feature of these models, goes from a low in Alaska of about 7 percent "seniors" to a high in Florida of almost 17 percent seniors.

Table 12-3 is a measure of the strength of the ultraviolet part of the sun that reaches the ground on average over the course of the entire year in the largest city of the state. This is the part known to cause sunburn or a suntan. The ultraviolet portion of sunlight is measured by the US government agency NOAA using satellite data over the entire United States to make a daily forecast of the intensity of this sun component. The UV Index is a daily forecast of the strength of ultraviolet reaching the ground during the middle of the day. The exact time is called "solar noon" for each location, around noon or 1 PM, depending on whether daylight savings time is in effect and where the city happens to be located within the time zone.

Many years ago, as I noted in earlier chapters, a NOAA scientist was kind enough to construct for me a yearly average from these daily numbers and these are what is presented here in Table 12-3. Pleased to find him after the passage of many years, he did the exercise for me once again, this time combining nine years together for years that were more recent. Both sets of numbers are very similar and I use whichever set works better.

Table 12-2 Older Age.
Percent Age 65 and Over in each state (2006).

State	%	State	%
Alaska	6.8	New Jersey	12.9
Utah	8.8	Kansas	12.9
Georgia	9.8	Oregon	12.9
Texas	9.9	Wisconsin	13.0
Colorado	10.0	New York	13.1
California	10.8	Oklahoma	13.2
Nevada	11.1	Nebraska	13.3
Idaho	11.5	Massachusetts	13.3
Washington	11.5	Vermont	13.3
Virginia	11.6	Missouri	13.3
Maryland	11.6	Connecticut	13.4
Illinois	12.0	Delaware	13.4
Minnesota	12.1	Alabama	13.4
Wyoming	12.2	Ohio	13.4
North Carolina	12.2	Montana	13.8
Louisiana	12.2	Rhode Island	13.9
District	12.3	Arkansas	13.9
New Mexico	12.4	Hawaii	14.0
New Hampshire	12.4	South Dakota	14.2
Indiana	12.4	North Dakota	14.6
Mississippi	12.4	Iowa	14.6
Michigan	12.5	Maine	14.6
Tennessee	12.7	Pennsylvania	15.2
Arizona	12.8	West Virginia	15.3
South Carolina	12.8	Florida	16.8
Kentucky	12.8		

Table 12-3 [ultra96] ultraviolet.
Average annual UVI (UV Index) score for the largest city in the state over the course of the year 1996.

Alaska	1.4	West Virginia	4.0
Washington	2.7	District	4.0
Vermont	2.9	Kentucky	4.1
Oregon	3.0	Missouri	4.1
Maine	3.1	Virginia	4.4
North Dakota	3.1	North Carolina	4.6
New Hampshire	3.2	Utah	4.7
Minnesota	3.2	Wyoming	4.7
Michigan	3.3	Kansas	4.7
Wisconsin	3.3	Arkansas	4.8
Massachusetts	3.3	Tennessee	4.8
Ohio	3.4	Colorado	4.9
Connecticut	3.4	Georgia	5.1
Rhode Island	3.4	Oklahoma	5.2
Illinois	3.5	South Carolina	5.3
South Dakota	3.5	Mississippi	5.5
Montana	3.5	Nevada	5.7
New York	3.6	Alabama	5.8
Indiana	3.7	Texas	5.9
Iowa	3.7	California	5.9
Nebraska	3.8	Louisiana	5.9
Pennsylvania	3.8	New Mexico	6.1
Maryland	3.9	Arizona	6.2
Delaware	3.9	Florida	6.9
New Jersey	3.9	Hawaii	9.6
Idaho	4.0		

My leniency in terms of the particular year of the data is partly due to availability but also because of a theoretical issue. We simply do not know which year of ultraviolet or the lack thereof would most strongly influence dying from ovarian cancer in around 2005.

To the best of my knowledge, this is the first research to link ultraviolet to ovarian cancer. Of course, it is the direction of this link which is a surprise. It is the insufficient strength of ultraviolet reaching the ground that is linked with this particular cancer rather than the opposite possibility that the sun is TOO strong. To characterize the result here as "counterintuitive" is not exactly right. Rather, the problem is that this finding conflicts with out current understanding. I hope to have more to say about this main finding later.

Looking at Table 12-3, these yearly averages for ultraviolet show the expected north-south pattern. Alaska, by far the most northern state, has a yearly UV Index (UVI) score of 1.4. Hawaii, the most southern state, has the highest score of 9.6. Of course, cloud cover and rain have an effect on this annual ultraviolet score.

Table 12-4 is the model for ovarian cancer death rates. It is our best attempt to explain the pattern of differences between the states in Table 12-1.

In the top box is Adjusted R Square, which is a summary number for how much of the pattern the model succeeds to explain. That is .726, 72.6 percent of the death rate pattern between the states.

Next, we jump to the bottom box to make sure that the two items are largely uncorrelated with each other. The preferred result of lack of correlation is sometimes difficult to achieve. Nevertheless, it is important to check it. An intercorrelation between the explanatory items, in this case, age and ultraviolet, might distort the results making them less reliable. Thankfully, in this case, both of these items are what I call "clean", largely uncorrelated. There are neither one nor two stars after the correlation numbers. This means that neither are correlated with each other to a solid enough degree to cause concern. Furthermore, the correlation numbers are very low.

The bottom line of this bottom box in Table 12-4 shows that both are correlated with the item in question, ovarian cancer deaths. This is interesting in its own way but secondary to the purpose of presenting these correlations which is to show that there is no large connection between the explanatory items used together in the model.

Table 12-4 The Ovarian Cancer Model:
The role of stronger ultraviolet (fewer deaths).

Model Summary

Model	R	R Square	Adjusted R Square	Std. Error of the Estimate
1	.859[a]	.737	.726	.5603

a. Predictors: (Constant), ULTRA96, AGE65IN6

Coefficients[a]

Model		Unstandardized Coefficients		Standardized Coefficients	t	Sig.
		B	Std. Error	Beta		
1	(Constant)	4.259	.639		6.662	.000
	AGE65IN6	.427	.048	.666	8.971	.000
	ULTRA96	-.482	.060	-.600	-8.080	.000

a. Dependent Variable: OVAR46AK

Correlations

		AGE65IN6	ULTRA96	OVAR46AK
AGE65IN6	Pearson Correlation	1	.084	.616**
	Sig. (2-tailed)	.	.560	.000
	N	51	51	51
ULTRA96	Pearson Correlation	.084	1	-.544**
	Sig. (2-tailed)	.560	.	.000
	N	51	51	51
OVAR46AK	Pearson Correlation	.616**	-.544**	1
	Sig. (2-tailed)	.000	.000	.
	N	51	51	51

**. Correlation is significant at the 0.01 level (2-tailed).

Now we can move to the main model in the middle box in Table 12-4. The end column shows both items with Sig .000, meaning that both connections with ovarian cancer are solid. This is reinforced in the second from the end "t" column where we like the value to be over 2. These values are very large at about 9 and 8. Solid.

Next is the middle column Beta in Table 12-4 which shows the size of each effect on deaths from ovarian cancer which can be compared directly to each other. It suggests that the some 73 percent of the pattern explained by this model is divided about equally between older age and ultraviolet with the effect of older age being a bit larger [.666 compared with (-).660].

In the Beta column, the unshown + sign indicates that the higher the percent of the population in a state that is age 65 or older, the MORE deaths from ovarian cancer in that state. Conversely, the minus sign in front of the .600 in the Beta column shows that the connection between ultraviolet and dying from ovarian cancer is "negative". The stronger the ultraviolet that reaches the ground in the largest city of the state, the fewer the deaths (per population size) from ovarian cancer in that state. Turning this around, the weaker the ultraviolet that reaches the ground, the more people who die from ovarian cancer.

These two effects, taken together, total one hundred percent of the portion that the model has succeeded to link with deaths from ovarian cancer. We know from the Adjusted R Square that the portion of the total pattern the model succeeds in capturing is a little less than three quarters. Of this, ultraviolet represents about 47.4 percent of that one hundred percent, a little less than half. We figured that out in this manner. From the Beta column eliminating the decimals and signs (+ and -): 666+600=1266. 600/1266=.4739 or about 47.4 percent.

We are more interested to know the size of the ultraviolet effect as a portion of the total explanation as this model only accounts for less than three quarters of that. To figure this, we want to know what the total of the two effects would be if they represented a hundred percent of the possible explanation. 1266/726=x/1000. 726x=1266000. x=1743.8016. Our ultraviolet effect 600/1743.8016=34.4 percent.

As a portion of the total explanation, the part captured in the model and the part not captured, ultraviolet represents 34.4% of that total explanation (of course a lower number). Thus, the strength of ultraviolet reaching the ground in the largest city of the state over the course of a given year (1996) accounts for a little more than a third of the pattern in deaths from ovarian cancer between states (during the years 2004, 2005 and 2006).

Next is the B column in Table 12-4 and these are the numbers of the actual equation summarizing the relationships in the model. While others use these numbers to specify the size of the effect of each item on ovarian cancer, we here use them to create a "best view" of ovarian cancer deaths.

The purpose of this exercise below is to create a more useful view of the pattern of dying from ovarian cancer across the country. Constructing this "best view" is subjective, based on my own idea about what seems most interesting to me and, hopefully, what other people might find interesting as well.

In Table 12-5, I present this "best view" of ovarian cancer death rates. I called it a "predicted" death rate which starts with the "actual" death rates by state in the given years, 2004-2006, from Table 12-1. The problem is that this actual set of numbers is meaningful only up to a point because there is no control for age.

While older age is a large item which helps to explain the pattern, it is something that is rather well known. Older people are more likely to die in general and more likely to die from cancer as well, generally speaking. Many of us would be interested to view the state list for ovarian cancer after accounting for that well known pattern. The big matter of differences between states in terms of how many older people there are is important for the main model. This is because only by accounting for this fact in the model can we explore what else might be connected with ovarian cancer.

For understanding the pattern of deaths from ovarian cancer, what seems more interesting than older age is the environmental item of the strength of the sun's ultraviolet reaching the ground. This is what we can view in the final list in Table 12-5.

Going back now to that middle box (in Table 12-4), the B column, we construct the equation using those numbers. For age whose effect we wish to minimize, we use the all-state average, the mean of all the numbers in Table 12-2 percent age 65. (That average percent of seniors in a state in 2006 happens to be 12.653 percent).

For our true interest, ultraviolet, we use the actual value for ultraviolet reaching the ground in the largest city of each state from Table 12-3. Thankfully, the software program (SPSS 11) calculates the solution for the equation for each state yielding the values in the final Table 12-5.

Table 12-5 [ovar461] ovarian 2004-2006 list.

Best view predicted death rate from ovarian cancer between 2004 and 2006 after first largely neutralizing the effect of older age (more deaths) in order to see the role of stronger ultraviolet (fewer deaths). As only ultraviolet varies, this ordering of states is the same as in Table 12-3 ultraviolet but reversed because stronger ultraviolet, fewer deaths from ovarian cancer.

Hawaii	5.03	Maryland	7.78
Florida	6.34	Delaware	7.78
Arizona	6.67	New Jersey	7.78
New Mexico	6.72	Nebraska	7.83
Texas	6.82	Pennsylvania	7.83
California	6.82	Indiana	7.88
Louisiana	6.82	Iowa	7.88
Alabama	6.87	New York	7.93
Nevada	6.91	Illinois	7.97
Mississippi	7.01	South Dakota	7.97
South Carolina	7.11	Montana	7.97
Oklahoma	7.16	Ohio	8.02
Georgia	7.20	Connecticut	8.02
Colorado	7.30	Rhode Island	8.02
Arkansas	7.35	Michigan	8.07
Tennessee	7.35	Wisconsin	8.07
Utah	7.40	Massachusetts	8.07
Wyoming	7.40	New Hampshire	8.12
Kansas	7.40	Minnesota	8.12
North Carolina	7.44	Maine	8.17
Virginia	7.54	North Dakota	8.17
Kentucky	7.69	Oregon	8.22
Missouri	7.69	Vermont	8.26
Idaho	7.73	Washington	8.36
West Virginia	7.73	Alaska	8.99
District	7.73		

The equation is as follows. 4.259 + (.427 * (times) mean value for age which is 12.653%) - (.482 * the annual UV Index value for each state from Table 12-3).

Let us take a look now at this "best view" of ovarian cancer death rates in Table 12-5. The first thing to note is that, after the effect of age is minimized, what remains to vary is only one item - ultraviolet. (The weaker the sun, the higher the death rate from ovarian cancer). For this reason, I wish to point to the obvious fact that the ordering of the states from lowest to highest death rate is the same (in reverse) as the ordering of the states in the ultraviolet list of Table 12-3.

In Table 12-5, Hawaii has the lowest ovarian cancer "predicted" death rate, about 5 deaths per hundred thousand people. This is because, in Table 12-3, Hawaii is the state with the strongest ultraviolet reaching the ground in Honolulu over the course of the year 1996. Conversely, the highest predicted death rate is in Alaska (about 9 deaths per hundred thousand) because, in Table 12-3 ultraviolet, Anchorage Alaska has the lowest annual strength of ultraviolet during 1996. These predicted rates in Table 12-5 are, of course, based on the actual death rates from ovarian cancer over the course of the years 2004-06.

I have little to add on the important topic of the link between cancer in general and older age. While I have no desire to minimize its importance, the topic is beyond my level of knowledge about the subject. For the task here, it was essential to have a "control" for age in the model before searching for other possible connections with ovarian cancer deaths.

In this simple, two item, model, what basically remains is one connection – between the strength of ultraviolet and dying from ovarian cancer. Of course, this remaining connection is environmental in nature, a focus here. The pattern revealed in this research of dying from ovarian cancer across the states in the American union (including the capital city of Washington DC), suggests a connection with ultraviolet.

Ultraviolet is one of three main constituents of sunlight, the part causing tanning (and burning). The stronger the ultraviolet that reaches the ground in the largest city of the state, the FEWER the people (women of course) who die from ovarian cancer (per hundred thousand people). The middle box in Table 12-4 with the main model shows this on the second line. The intensity of ultraviolet reaching the ground is solidly connected in a negative direction with dying from ovarian cancer in 2004-06. Weaker ultraviolet reaching the ground, more deaths from ovarian cancer.

How are we to interpret this result which many will find surprising? First we can try to "falsify" the result. Ultraviolet reaching the ground varies closely with latitude. Such is the case even though the numbers for latitude INCREASE as we move north (in the Northern hemisphere) while those for ultraviolet DECREASE as we move north. The strength of ultraviolet as represented in these annual UV Index numbers decreases as we travel away from the equator. This is because sunlight hits the ground more on an angle the more north we go.

Because so many environmental factors vary with latitude, how can we be sure that it is ultraviolet specifically rather other items that may vary. These include air temperature, patterns of cosmic radiation, cloudiness itself, etc. which might vary together with ultraviolet. A drawback of this research method is that we can never be completely sure. We become more confident by testing the option of ultraviolet in competition with alternatives many of which I have numbers for and have done. Ultraviolet comes out strongest.

This connection between weaker ultraviolet and higher death rates from ovarian cancer does not prove that insufficient exposure to ultraviolet is what CAUSES this cancer. This kind of study is unable to prove causation. Nevertheless, it provides evidence for the possibility that the lack of strong enough ultraviolet MIGHT be causally involved with the development of ovarian cancer which leads to death from this disease.

Another question involves the nature of sunlight. How do we know it is ultraviolet specifically that is connected with ovarian cancer rather than other parts of the solar spectrum. These include the large component of heat energy (infrared) as well as visible light. While the ultraviolet part of the solar spectrum has the strongest energy, it is only about five percent of total sunlight.

In general, the different components of sunlight are highly correlated with each other. Might it not be possible that it is another component of sunlight that is responsible for this statistical connection?

One alternative idea I have tested is the "total solar energy" which reaches a solar collector on the ground in the largest city of the state. This, however, is unconnected with the pattern of ovarian cancer deaths.

The success of ultraviolet specifically could be the result of the sophistication of the UV Index measurement compared to other measurements for sunlight. The UV Index (NOAA) converts the absolute energy of ultraviolet reaching the ground to a form which captures its specific effect on human skin. Added to this is the satellite data on weather conditions which affect the prediction for how intense the ultraviolet part of sunlight reaching the ground will be on the following day.

Of course, it is in the nature of this "correlational" research that it is always possible that the item specified in the model might actually be merely linked with the genuine "causal" agent which might be something different. Nevertheless, from the testing done here, the best evidence suggests that ultraviolet itself is the strongest choice for explaining this pattern of deaths from ovarian cancer (given the limitations discussed here).

Perhaps we can speculate a little on how the lack of strong sunlight reaching the ground might be linked with dying from ovarian cancer. It seems somewhat reasonable to assume that we are talking here about a person's exposure to ultraviolet which occurs when that portion of the sun is at its strongest, around midday.

Of course, this research is not capable of measuring exposure directly. It would be virtually impossible to do in this kind of study given its extreme macro nature. It is as if we are looking at the United States from "space", from a point so far up that it is outside the planet's atmosphere, observing this pattern of increasing deaths from ovarian cancer as we go from south to north.

One possibility is that such exposure to midday sun varies from place to place. While this might be true, it is a complicated matter to think through given that so many people are indoors in the middle of the day working in offices. While more people might be outside in warmer weather, it is also reasonable to think that many might avoid the heat (or humidity). They may prefer to be indoors being adjusted to the comfortable conditions of air conditioning. Then there is the matter of sunscreen and perhaps make-up blocking the skin from direct exposure to sunlight.

There is a key point which must raise questions about the idea that exposure to sunlight must vary from place to place as an explanation for the finding here. Such variation in exposure to sunlight must vary systematically in a pattern that would fit this northern pattern. It strikes me as implausible that, as we travel north, fewer people go outside in the middle of the day.

The idea of differences in exposure is an important enough matter to merit an additional test. Sun AVOIDANCE might be greater with higher education, as it is the current recommendation of health experts. Weather conditions such as humidity and dew point might also keep people inside at the proper time of day, not to mention outdoor temperatures.

We can test these various items using our final model here from Table 12-4. In the test (model not shown), while the original items of age and ultraviolet continue to be significantly related to dying from ovarian cancer, none of the other four items come out as related as the results are not statistically significant (at the .01 level). These include education [sumcolig], humidity [humidity], dew point during the month of June [dewjune] and average temperature (from 1971-2000)[teme7100].

We can roughly conclude, then, that there is no connection between dying from ovarian cancer and levels of education or the three weather variations which we presume might affect patterns of being outside during the middle of the day. This reinforces my thinking that the matter of variations in exposure to sunlight is unlikely to conform to a systematic pattern that would fit the result here - that the more north we go, the more people die from ovarian cancer.

Thankfully, there is another idea which might work better as an explanation. While exposure to sunlight hitting the skin must somehow be involved in the posited biological effect which results in fewer deaths from ovarian cancer, the explanation must lie in a change in the sunlight itself.

Sunlight together with its ultraviolet portion changes as we travel north. It gets weaker. This is what must result in more deaths from ovarian cancer. It is the weaker intensity of ultraviolet that must be the "culprit".

According to my current understanding, even exposure to ultraviolet from the sun might be no guarantee for warding off ovarian cancer, even though it is the right time of day (midday) and without sunscreen (or makeup). If a person lives too far north where the sun is weaker, whatever exposure there is might not be sufficient. This is because the sun itself, its ultraviolet portion, might not be strong enough to have its posited protective effect.

Chapter 13. Uterine Cancer Linked with Air Pollution, Insufficiently Strong Ultraviolet - as well as with Visiting the Dentist!

For death from uterine cancer, I end up presenting two models instead of one on the assumption that the strange result in the second model might be too important to ignore.

As is our pattern, we start with death rates from uterine cancer by state, using, this time, the most recent numbers (at the time of this writing) - deaths during the years 2012, 2013 and 2014. This list is on Table 13-1. Please note that, as with the other exclusively female cancers, the death rates are presented as a portion of the entire population including women as well as men. The actual death rate among women only, then, is around double, assuming women are about half the population. I decided to present it this way for two reasons. The numbers in this form seem more reliable and they are also easier to compare with other cancers.

For uterine cancer, the death rates range from a low in Alaska of 2.2 deaths per hundred thousand people, to a high in Delaware of 5.3 deaths. Looking over the list of states in Table 13-1, California is on the low side, Florida on the high side with New York and New Jersey very high. Of course, the purpose of constructing a model of these numbers is to use these differences between places to learn about this cancer – with what it might be linked in the environment and in the area of lifestyle.

Once again, the usual caveat applies that we are unable to definitively conclude from this type of research what actually causes uterine cancer. Instead, uncovering these connections can only provide evidence to support the possibility that these factors might be involved in explaining deaths from this cancer.

Largely following the format from other cancers, I will summarize how the presentation will appear. First, I identify and discuss the four items that are part of the models. (For uterine cancer, there are two separate models instead of one typically). Then I present the first model including the "best view" list of "predicted" death rates to gain a clearer understanding of the list of states in a form that is most useful. After that, I present the second model and the "best view" list of states based on that model. While I could have decided to combine together the main findings into one model, instead, I chose two separate models for a technical reason - to maintain the pristine solidness of the connections in each.

Table 13-1 [uter1214] uterine 2012-2014.

Average annual death rate from uterine cancer between 2012 and 2014 by state (per hundred thousand population including both women and men).

State	Rate	State	Rate
		Nebraska	3.8
Alaska	2.2	Montana	3.8
Nevada	2.5	South Carolina	3.9
Utah	2.5	North Carolina	3.9
Colorado	2.7	Missouri	3.9
Wyoming	2.8	Connecticut	3.9
Texas	2.9	New Hampshire	3.9
North Dakota	2.9	Oregon	3.9
Alabama	3.0	Florida	4.0
Arizona	3.1	Massachusetts	4.0
Oklahoma	3.1	Wisconsin	4.1
Arkansas	3.1	Indiana	4.3
Hawaii	3.2	Illinois	4.4
New Mexico	3.2	Ohio	4.4
Mississippi	3.2	Michigan	4.4
California	3.4	Maine	4.4
Louisiana	3.4	West Virginia	4.5
Tennessee	3.4	Rhode Island	4.6
Idaho	3.4	Maryland	4.7
Georgia	3.5	Vermont	4.8
Kentucky	3.5	Iowa	4.9
Minnesota	3.5	New York	4.9
Washington	3.5	New Jersey	5.0
South Dakota	3.6	Pennsylvania	5.1
Kansas	3.7	District	5.2
Virginia	3.7	Delaware	5.3

The four items linked with uterine cancer death rates are as follows: First is our familiar age 65 and over (more deaths). Second is a less common one - particle air pollution (more deaths). Third is weaker ultraviolet from the sun (more deaths). Fourth is visiting the dentist (more who visited, MORE deaths) - to my considerable shock.

Age 65 is found in Table 13-2, the percent of the population in the state that is age 65 and over, which I often call "seniors". This is for the year 2006. Alaska has the fewest seniors as a percent of the population, about 7 percent. Florida has the largest percent seniors, about 17 percent.

This is the first cancer model since breast cancer for which air pollution is a large and solid enough item to make it into the final model. Government scientists, combining state and federal employees, have a network of air pollution monitors to follow several kinds of air pollution. The most common of these are ozone air pollution, a gas, and particle air pollution (2.5 microns), microscopic pieces of dirt (carbon) in the air so small that you cannot see them with the naked eye. This kind of air pollution is known generally as particle pollution or by the more technical term particulate matter 2.5 microns.

The airnow.gov site, with rare exceptions, provides real time readings for these two kinds of air pollution in large cities (where the problem is usually worse). These readings are aggregated to daily averages and then yearly averages for small areas of many large cities. It is these numbers that appear in Table 13-3 [pmmetro], one of several versions of yearly averages in the downtown areas of the largest city of the state. I believe these yearly averages in Table 13-3 are for the year 2007.

I selected for this uterine cancer model this particular version of particle pollution numbers (and not ozone) because it worked best in the process of model building, came out most largely and solidly linked with the pattern of uterine cancer deaths across the states.

Typically, health work correlating air pollution to various diseases, death rates or incidence rates (having the illness), is done in research that is far more "micro" - working with county or city level health data. In a somewhat unusual macro analysis such as this, I use the downtown air pollution information in the largest city of the state to represent the entire state. This is despite the fact that air quality varies, improves typically, as we gain distance from the center of the city.

Table 13-2 Older Age.
Percent Age 65 and Over in each state (2006).

State	%	State	%
Alaska	6.8	Kentucky	12.8
Utah	8.8	New Jersey	12.9
Georgia	9.8	Kansas	12.9
Texas	9.9	Oregon	12.9
Colorado	10.0	Wisconsin	13.0
California	10.8	New York	13.1
Nevada	11.1	Oklahoma	13.2
Idaho	11.5	Nebraska	13.3
Washington	11.5	Massachusetts	13.3
Virginia	11.6	Vermont	13.3
Maryland	11.6	Missouri	13.3
Illinois	12.0	Connecticut	13.4
Minnesota	12.1	Delaware	13.4
Wyoming	12.2	Alabama	13.4
North Carolina	12.2	Ohio	13.4
Louisiana	12.2	Montana	13.8
District	12.3	Rhode Island	13.9
New Mexico	12.4	Arkansas	13.9
New Hampshire	12.4	Hawaii	14.0
Indiana	12.4	South Dakota	14.2
Mississippi	12.4	North Dakota	14.6
Michigan	12.5	Iowa	14.6
Tennessee	12.7	Maine	14.6
Arizona	12.8	Pennsylvania	15.2
South Carolina	12.8	West Virginia	15.3
		Florida	16.8

Table 13-3 [pmmetro] particulate matter in the metropolitan area. Average annual particle air pollution (particulate matter 2.5 microns) in the largest city of the state.

State	Value	State	Value
Wyoming	4.9	Rhode Island	13.0
Hawaii	5.8	South Carolina	13.1
Alaska	5.9	Arkansas	13.4
Montana	7.4	North Carolina	13.7
North Dakota	7.9	Mississippi	13.8
Idaho	8.0	Kentucky	13.8
Oregon	9.1	Missouri	14.4
Florida	9.4	Texas	14.7
Vermont	10.1	Delaware	15.3
Oklahoma	10.2	Tennessee	15.4
New Hampshire	10.3	New York	15.8
South Dakota	10.4	New Jersey	16.0
Colorado	10.6	West Virginia	16.1
New Mexico	10.6	Pennsylvania	16.1
Nevada	10.7	Virginia	16.2
Washington	10.7	District	16.2
Iowa	10.7	Indiana	16.3
Nebraska	11.0	Illinois	16.8
Kansas	11.2	Maryland	16.8
Arizona	11.3	Connecticut	16.9
Louisiana	12.0	Alabama	17.4
Minnesota	12.0	Ohio	17.6
Utah	12.3	Georgia	17.7
Massachusetts	12.3	Michigan	19.1
Wisconsin	12.7	California	22.1
Maine	12.7		

I decided on this unconventional macro analysis in the belief that, despite the rough nature of the analysis, air quality in the largest city might, nevertheless, serve as a window to general air quality in the state as a whole. The successful result here shows a connection between higher air pollution in the downtown of the largest city and higher death rates from uterine cancer across the entire state. It appears to confirm the usefulness of this unconventional approach.

Looking now at Table 13-3 for particle pollution by state (in the downtown of the largest city), the lowest level is in Wyoming followed by Hawaii and Alaska. Not surprisingly to me is the place of New York (number 37 best out of 51) and New Jersey (number 38 best out of 51). California does the worst at number 51 "best", having the highest particle pollution in the downtown of their largest city, Los Angeles, (of course). Lastly, reflecting my own interest in places, is Florida, which does quite well, with the 8th lowest level of particle air pollution (based on Miami).

Moving now to another environmental item, ultraviolet is in Table 13-4. The federal government agency NOAA has an excellent program measuring the ultraviolet portion of the sun which reaches the ground. It makes a daily prediction during the previous afternoon for what the ultraviolet intensity will be the following day at "solar noon", around 12 or 1 o'clock.

As I mentioned earlier, a kind hearted scientist aggregated these numbers from daily to yearly averages for each of my big cities (which largely coincide with the cities measured by NOAA) creating for me a yearly average during the year 1996. To my knowledge, this exercise was special for the research here.

The same scientist redid this for me a second time many many years later. In this second effort, he used a series of more recent years. This second attempt turned out to be surprisingly similar to the 1996 yearly averages (when I tested the correlation between the two sets of numbers). I used the 1996 numbers here because they linked most strongly with the pattern of deaths from uterine cancer.

There is little doubt that this government effort to monitor ultraviolet was launched due to the consensus belief that ultraviolet, the tanning part of the sun, can be dangerous and harmful. For this reason, I must be careful to make clear that neither the agency nor its employees endorse the result here which would probably be considered unexpected. Of course, I am talking about the finding soon to be presented that it is lower (rather than higher) intensities of ultraviolet that are connected with more deaths from uterine cancer.

As I have written elsewhere, the strength of ultraviolet reaching the ground is highly correlated with the other two major portions of sunlight, the majority part being infrared radiation or heat, and the other large part, visible light. While I have a different kind of measure of total solar radiation in a city, it is ultraviolet that links most strongly and clearly with the pattern of deaths from uterine cancer (weaker ultraviolet, more deaths).

For measuring the strength of the other two portions of sunlight, I have had to improvise using the available data I have found. Average annual air temperature over the last 30 years is perhaps a good measure for infrared even though it is indirect (in that the heat portion of sunlight indirectly heats the air). I know that ultraviolet works better than average air temperature in a state.

An independent measure for the strength of visible light might be a problem. Given the strong correlation between the strength of the three components, we cannot be certain that it is the ultraviolet portion specifically that links most closely to uterine cancer deaths. Perhaps it is the insufficient intensity of the light portion that is, instead, the key. Given the available data, however, the best evidence suggests that it is ultraviolet specifically (even though we cannot be entirely certain).

During a later read, I decided to add the following additional thought. Maybe the numbers for ultraviolet work best because they are different from other ways to measure the intensity of sunlight that I have tested. In creating the UV Index, the scientists convert the actual measurement of ultraviolet reaching the ground to a form which takes into consideration its impact on human skin. This could partly account for the unusual success here of the UV Index compared with other ways to measure the intensity of sunlight such as "total solar radiation", tested here with the items called [solarflat] and [suninsol].

Lastly, I should point out that these UV Index numbers are a yearly average. They include the strength of ultraviolet for each place not only in summer when it is highest but also in winter when it is lowest. The July value, at the height of the summer, is, of course, higher than this annual average.

Looking now at Table 13-4 ultraviolet, Alaska has the lowest yearly level and Hawaii has the highest, both states being in their own "league" of low and high. Looking again at the high section, not surprisingly, a few other large states come out "high" for the sun's ultraviolet radiation reaching the ground. These include Florida, Arizona, California and Texas. Little Rhode Island is quite low for strong sun at number-12-lowest of 51 "states".

We can now move to the number four connection with uterine cancer - visiting the dentist - in Table 13-7. (Even though I mention it now, I placed this list several pages forward in the text due to its connection with the second model). This is the percent of a representative sample of state respondents in a health survey who said they visited the dentist in the past year. It goes from a low in West Virginia of about 53 percent who said they had visited the dentist to a high in Connecticut of about 79 percent who said they saw the dentist.

Results for this item are presented in a separate second model for death rates from uterine cancer. To repeat, strangely, the more people who said they visited the dentist, the more women there were who died of uterine cancer.

Being already familiar with the items that came out as linked with the pattern of deaths from uterine cancer across the states, we can now turn to the first of the two models. These models are attempts to "explain" or account for the pattern of differences in cancer deaths between the states. Later we will develop a "best view" list of predicted death rates which we will construct from the models which result.

The first uterine cancer model appears in Table 13-5. First, we skip to the bottom box which shows the "zero order" correlations between the items. There are two reasons for this review. The first is to ensure that there is no troubling degree of connectedness between the items which violate the rules of the method. The second reason is the feared consequence when this happens – invalid results which can mislead us.

Table 13-4 [ultra96] ultraviolet 1996.
Average annual ultraviolet reaching the ground at solar noon when it is strongest in the largest city of the state during the year 1996. This is the UVI (UV Index) value over an entire year from NOAA.

State	UVI	State	UVI
Alaska	1.4	West Virginia	4.0
Washington	2.7	District	4.0
Vermont	2.9	Kentucky	4.1
Oregon	3.0	Missouri	4.1
North Dakota	3.1	Virginia	4.4
Maine	3.1	North Carolina	4.6
New Hampshire	3.2	Wyoming	4.7
Minnesota	3.2	Kansas	4.7
Massachusetts	3.3	Utah	4.7
Wisconsin	3.3	Arkansas	4.8
Michigan	3.3	Tennessee	4.8
Rhode Island	3.4	Colorado	4.9
Connecticut	3.4	Georgia	5.1
Ohio	3.4	Oklahoma	5.2
Montana	3.5	South Carolina	5.3
South Dakota	3.5	Mississippi	5.5
Illinois	3.5	Nevada	5.7
New York	3.6	Alabama	5.8
Iowa	3.7	Louisiana	5.9
Indiana	3.7	Texas	5.9
Nebraska	3.8	California	5.9
Pennsylvania	3.8	New Mexico	6.1
Delaware	3.9	Arizona	6.2
New Jersey	3.9	Florida	6.9
Maryland	3.9	Hawaii	9.6
Idaho	4.0		

Table 13-5 The Uterine Cancer Model: the role of particle air pollution (more deaths) as well as stronger ultraviolet in sunlight (fewer deaths).

Model Summary

Model	R	R Square	Adjusted R Square	Std. Error of the Estimate
1	.766[a]	.587	.560	.5018

a. Predictors: (Constant), ULTRA96, PMMETRO, AGE65IN6

Coefficients[a]

Model		Unstandardized Coefficients		Standardized Coefficients	t	Sig.
		B	Std. Error	Beta		
1	(Constant)	.433	.633		.684	.497
	AGE65IN6	.247	.043	.546	5.800	.000
	PMMETRO	8.824E-02	.020	.424	4.516	.000
	ULTRA96	-.211	.054	-.371	-3.944	.000

a. Dependent Variable: UTER1214

Correlations

		AGE65IN6	PMMETRO	ULTRA96	UTER1214
AGE65IN6	Pearson Correlation	1	-.018	.084	.507**
	Sig. (2-tailed)	.	.899	.560	.000
	N	51	51	51	51
PMMETRO	Pearson Correlation	-.018	1	-.042	.430**
	Sig. (2-tailed)	.899	.	.769	.002
	N	51	51	51	51
ULTRA96	Pearson Correlation	.084	-.042	1	-.344*
	Sig. (2-tailed)	.560	.769	.	.014
	N	51	51	51	51
UTER1214	Pearson Correlation	.507**	.430**	-.344*	1
	Sig. (2-tailed)	.000	.002	.014	.
	N	51	51	51	51

**. Correlation is significant at the 0.01 level (2-tailed).
*. Correlation is significant at the 0.05 level (2-tailed).

The bottom box shows the items happily free of intercorrelation with no stars (above and to the right). (Such stars would have suggested correlations that are statistically significant). Furthermore, the actual size of the values in the correlation boxes are low. While in the area, we also glance at the bottom row and see that the connections with our item of focus, deaths from uterine cancer, are there for all, mainly for age and particle pollution [pmmetro].

Next, we jump to the top box and see that the Adjusted R Square is .560. This is on the low side. The model as a whole explains 56% of the pattern of differences in death rates between states.

Finally, we arrive to the first model itself in the middle box of Table 13-5. On the right side, we see a Sig (t) of .000 for all three items, the best score, with the actual numbers on which this score is based in the next column to the left: "t". Needing values of 2 or more for statistical significance, these numbers are much higher, about 6, 5 and 4. This suggests that the results are solid.

We check statistical significance on the theoretical assumption that we are dealing with a sample of deaths from a larger population. As I mention earlier, one could also argue the reverse. After all, we are dealing with all deaths, as best we know, (over this three years period) from uterine cancer in the United States rather than just a sample of them.

Nevertheless, we could still imagine that these deaths (in the form of deaths rates listed in Table 13-1) are a subset of deaths from other years and perhaps even other places. After all, we are hoping to use these US state death numbers to learn about uterine cancer in general. For this reason, the numbers in this specific model CAN be seen as a sample of sorts.

While such testing of statistical significance may or may not really be necessary, I like to employ this test as a way to assess the "solidness" of the relationships stated. I use the cutoff of .01 as opposed to .05 employing this more difficult test as an additional way to make sure that the stated connections with uterine cancer deaths are solid.

As I discuss earlier, this by itself, does not solve the other inherent weaknesses of this correlational research. This includes the possibility that the selected items in the model might not be the "true" connections but rather items highly linked with something else entirely. For this threat, we build an argument that it is "this" item rather than "that". This includes testing alternatives to see which works best, links most cleanly and powerfully with the matter at hand, dying from uterine cancer.

For building this final model, I have first done such testing by building many earlier models along the way, sometimes in the tens of models, testing, culling, to see which items are the most successful, linked most cleanly and powerfully with uterine cancer.

The core of the main model in Table 13-5 is in the middle Beta column (of the middle box). These numbers can be compared in size with each other. Together they represent a hundred percent of the three items identified in the model (but only 56% of the total explanation).

To identify how this explained part of the pattern is divided up, we add together the three numbers (ignoring the decimals and direction signs): (546+424+371=1341). We then divide each by the total: older age=546/1341=.407, 40.7 percent of the explained portion. Particle pollution [pmmetro] = 424/1341=.316 or 31.6 percent. Ultraviolet [ultra96]=371/1341=27.7 percent.

As a portion of the entire explanation, the part identified in the model, and the part not identified, still unknown, these percents will be much smaller. We will make that calculation now given that this description, more modest in size, is probably the most meaningful one.

The combined total of the three identified items is 1341 which represents 56 percent (based on the Adjusted R Square). We now want to know what the total would be if we had 100 percent of the explanation. 1341/.560=x/1. 1341=.560x. x=2394.643. We can divide each beta value into this larger number and we will see the total value of each item identified in the model as a portion of the total explanation. This includes both the part identified in the model and the part not identified.

Older age is 546/2394.643=.228 or 22.8 percent of the total explanation, the largest finding. Second is particle air pollution [pmmetro] 424/2394.643=.177 or 17.7 percent of the total explanation. Lastly is ultraviolet [ultra96] which is 371/2394.643=.1549 or 15.5 percent of the total explanation.

This is perhaps the most meaningful number which captures the size of this research result to come out of this model on uterine cancer. Ultraviolet explains 15.5 percent of the pattern of difference in death rates between states. Particle air pollution explains a slightly larger amount of the total explanation, 17.7 percent.

The actual equation of the model is found in the middle box of Table 13-5, in the B column, the most left set of numbers. While these numbers can be used to specify an exact unit change of one item leading to a unit change in death rates from uterine cancer, we here use the actual equation for another purpose. We will build a new "best view" list of states and their "predicted" death rates to develop what we think is the most meaningful look at the pattern.

To do this, we strongly minimize the impact of older age, a connection which is powerful due to its link with dying from cancer. Yes, more women die in states where there are more older people as a portion of the population. We need this in the model in order to look further at other factors.

We control for age by building the equation using the numbers in the B column but instead of using the actual percent age 65 listed in Table 13-2, we plug in the mean for all the 51 states on that list which happens to be about thirteen percent (12.653).

For this best view list, because there are two environmental items of interest which affect the pattern of uterine cancer deaths between states, we allow both to "vary". We plug in the actual values for each state found for particle air pollution in Table 13-3 and found for ultraviolet in Table 13-4. To repeat, what will result is our constructed best view which first minimizes the effect of older age so we can get a better look at the effect of the environment on deaths from this cancer.

We now turn to those numbers in the B column of the second box in Table 13-5 and construct that equation which is a numerical representation of the result that is an attempt to explain the pattern in the original death rate list for uterine cancer in Table 13-1.

Below is that equation using the average value for age 65 for all the states but using the actual state values for the two environmental items of particle air pollution and ultraviolet reaching the ground in sunlight. .433 + (.247 * (times) the average all-states value for age 65 12.653) + (.08824, another way of writing the number, * [pmmetro], the actual state value for air pollution, - (.211 * [ultra96], the value for each state.

The statistical software (SPSS 11) allows us to easily solve this equation for each state resulting in the list in Table 13-6 Predicted death rate from uterine cancer per hundred thousand people (women and men) based on actual deaths between 2012 and 2014. As the effect of older age is held constant, the ordering of states reflects mainly the interplay of the role of air pollution and ultraviolet, with air pollution being slightly larger in size.

Looking now at Table 13-6, the "best view", we see that the state with the lowest death rates from uterine cancer is Hawaii. This is due to a combination of two results. Firstly, Hawaii has the second lowest level of particle air pollution according to Table 13-3. Secondly, Hawaii is the state with the very highest intensity of ultraviolet reaching the ground over the course of the year in Table 13-4 (end of list). This is largely due to its very southern location, close to the equator, and much farther south than Florida.

Speaking of Florida, it comes out in Table 13-6 as the state with the second lowest level of uterine cancer deaths because of ITS two characteristics. First is Florida's reasonably low level of air pollution in Table 13-3, 8th lowest of 51 states. Second is Florida's ultraviolet, the second highest (strongest) ultraviolet of all the states [according to Table 13-4 (after Hawaii)].

I can pick other states of interest to me looking over Table 13-6 a bit more. Rhode Island, as well as New Jersey and New York are toward the bottom of the list (more deaths) because of their combination of high particle air pollution in Table 13-3 (linked with higher uterine cancer death rates) combined with not so strong ultraviolet reaching the ground in Providence, Newark and New York City, all in the top half of the list in Table 13-4.

This table 13-6 is the "best view" of death rates from this cancer because it reduces the effect of older age. Keep in mind, however, that it only accounts for the portion of the pattern we succeeded here in capturing in the model, 56 percent (the Adjusted R Square in the top box of Table 13-5).

Ordinarily, I would stop the chapter on uterine cancer right here. Instead, I wish to present a second model for this cancer similar to the first in that the first two items are the same, age and air pollution. The third item is changed, however, from ultraviolet - to a new item - visiting the dentist. I decided to include it partly because the result is so counterintuitive that I figured it might be important. If correct, it is my hope that a different person might be able to figure it out better than I can.

In keeping with the pattern of all the models, I refer readers to the lists for the first two items, age and air pollution, from earlier in the chapter. These are in Table 13-2 older age, and Table 13-3 particle air pollution. Also relevant, of course, are the starting death rate numbers for uterine cancer in Table 13-1.

Now we can take a look at the new item which can be found in Table 13-7 dentist [dentlvis]. This is the percent of the state population that visited the dentist over the past year. It goes from a low in West Virginia of some 53 percent who saw the dentist to a high in Connecticut of 79 percent who said they saw the dentist.

This second uterine cancer model can be found in Table 13-8. We start by looking at the bottom box and we notice that the three items are "clean" in that they are largely uncorrelated with each other.

Glancing down at the connection with the item of interest, deaths from uterine cancer, all are correlated. As before, the first two items are linked with two stars, at the .01 level of statistical significance and the third with one star, the .05 level, not as good. Visiting the dentist is somewhat linked in a "zero order" correlation with dying from this cancer. These zero order correlations are only secondary in importance, of course, because we wait to see the final model above (in Table 13-8).

Next we turn to the top box in Table 13-8 and see the Adjusted R Square of the model is .562 meaning that this model explains 56.2 percent of the pattern reflected in the original numbers in Table 13-1. This is almost identical in size with the first model. It is actually possible to combine all the findings into one model but I felt it technically stronger to present each separately.

The relative size of each item is quite similar to the first model with older age playing a somewhat less prominent role as the only apparent difference.

Like in the last uterine cancer model, to learn the relative importance of each item out of 100 percent of the portion that the model succeeds in explaining, we add the three numbers (without decimals and signs) and use this number as the denominator to find the portion that can be attributed to each item. 539+422+373=1334.

Age is 539/1334=.404 or 40.4 percent of the explained portion. Air pollution [pmmetro] is 422/1334=.316 or 31.6 percent of the explained portion of the pattern. Finally, visiting the dentist [dentlvis] is 373/1334=.2796 or 28.0 percent of this explained portion.

Table 13-6 [uteruvl] uterine ultraviolet list.
Best view predicted death rate from uterine cancer per hundred thousand people (women and men) based on actual deaths between 2012 and 2014, average annual. The effect of older age is set aside in order to have a clearer look at the two environmental items: particle air pollution (more deaths) and stronger ultraviolet (fewer deaths).

Hawaii	2.04	Alabama	3.87
Florida	2.93	Tennessee	3.90
Wyoming	3.00	Kentucky	3.91
New Mexico	3.21	Washington	3.93
Arizona	3.25	Minnesota	3.94
Nevada	3.30	Massachusetts	3.95
Oklahoma	3.36	Missouri	3.96
Louisiana	3.37	Wisconsin	3.98
Idaho	3.42	Rhode Island	3.99
Colorado	3.46	Maine	4.02
Montana	3.47	Georgia	4.04
Kansas	3.55	Virginia	4.06
South Carolina	3.60	Delaware	4.09
North Dakota	3.60	West Virginia	4.13
Texas	3.61	District	4.14
Mississippi	3.62	New Jersey	4.15
Utah	3.65	Pennsylvania	4.18
Iowa	3.72	New York	4.19
Nebraska	3.73	Indiana	4.22
Arkansas	3.73	Maryland	4.22
Oregon	3.73	California	4.26
South Dakota	3.74	Illinois	4.30
Alaska	3.78	Connecticut	4.33
New Hampshire	3.79	Ohio	4.39
North Carolina	3.80	Michigan	4.55
Vermont	3.84		

Table 13-7 [dentlvis] dental visits.
Percent of state population that visited the dentist over the past year.

State	%	State	%
West Virginia	53.1	Arizona	68.9
Mississippi	57.1	California	69.0
Oklahoma	57.8	Colorado	69.2
Arkansas	58.5	Oregon	70.2
Louisiana	58.9	Pennsylvania	70.2
Nevada	59.2	Illinois	70.6
Alabama	60.1	Iowa	70.8
Kentucky	60.2	Alaska	71.1
Missouri	60.8	Delaware	71.1
Texas	61.7	New York	71.2
North Dakota	62.9	District	71.4
New Mexico	64.2	Vermont	71.7
Montana	64.3	Maryland	71.9
Georgia	64.7	Nebraska	72.4
Wyoming	65.4	Utah	72.9
Idaho	65.7	New Hampshire	72.9
Indiana	66.6	Minnesota	72.9
Ohio	66.6	Virginia	73.1
South Dakota	66.9	New Jersey	73.6
Kansas	67.0	Rhode Island	75.4
South Carolina	67.0	Wisconsin	75.5
North Carolina	67.1	Massachusetts	75.9
Maine	67.2	Hawaii	77.0
Tennessee	67.5	Michigan	78.0
Washington	67.9	Connecticut	79.1
Florida	68.8		

Table 13-8 The Second Uterine Cancer Model with Dentist.
The role of going to the dentist (more deaths).

Model Summary

Model	R	R Square	Adjusted R Square	Std. Error of the Estimate
1	.767[a]	.588	.562	.5011

a. Predictors: (Constant), DENTLVIS, PMMETRO, AGE65IN6

Coefficients[a]

Model		Unstandardized Coefficients		Standardized Coefficients	t	Sig.
		B	Std. Error	Beta		
1	(Constant)	-3.699	1.037		-3.565	.001
	AGE65IN6	.244	.042	.539	5.741	.000
	PMMETRO	8.791E-02	.020	.422	4.505	.000
	DENTLVIS	4.806E-02	.012	.373	3.966	.000

a. Dependent Variable: UTER1214

Correlations

		AGE65IN6	PMMETRO	DENTLVIS	UTER1214
AGE65IN6	Pearson Correlation	1	-.018	-.065	.507**
	Sig. (2-tailed)	.	.899	.653	.000
	N	51	51	51	51
PMMETRO	Pearson Correlation	-.018	1	.046	.430**
	Sig. (2-tailed)	.899	.	.749	.002
	N	51	51	51	51
DENTLVIS	Pearson Correlation	-.065	.046	1	.357*
	Sig. (2-tailed)	.653	.749	.	.010
	N	51	51	51	51
UTER1214	Pearson Correlation	.507**	.430**	.357*	1
	Sig. (2-tailed)	.000	.002	.010	.
	N	51	51	51	51

**. Correlation is significant at the 0.01 level (2-tailed).
*. Correlation is significant at the 0.05 level (2-tailed).

Of course, because the model explains a little more than half the pattern, the relative size of these items will shrink further as a portion of the entire explanation, the part explained here by the model and the part left unexplained. It is worthwhile to specify these smaller numbers as well, a more realistic conclusion about what we have accomplished here in terms of the total explanation.

If the total of the three numbers in the Beta column of Table 13-8 comes to 1334 which represents 56.2 percent of the explanation, what is this total in terms of the whole explanation? $1334/56.2=x/100$. $56.2x=133400$. $x=2373.665$.

Age is then $539/2373.665=.227$ or 22.7 percent of the total explanation. Older age accounts for a little over a fifth of the total explanation of the pattern of death rates from uterine cancer in the original list in Table 13-1.

Air pollution is $422/2373.665=.117778$ or 11.8 percent of the total explanation of the pattern in Table 13-1. Visiting the dentist is $373/2373.665=.157$ or 15.7 percent of the total pattern reflected in the original uterine death rate numbers from Table 13-1.

Now for the shocker if you haven't already picked up on it. I almost missed it myself. Going to the dentist is also present in some other cancer models and it was always a good thing. The higher the portion of the population that said they visited the dentist over the past year, the lower the death rate from this cancer and that. I gave this a broad interpretation assuming first that visiting the dentist involved doing healthful things that might help to prevent cancer. I further assumed that dental visits might provide education and motivation that improved daily oral care at home – which might involve flossing and brushing (and perhaps other behaviors).

In this model for uterine cancer, however, the sign, the direction of the effect, is in the OPPOSITE direction. This is obvious in the middle box of Table 13-8. There is no negative sign in front of the number for dentist in the Beta column .373. This means that the relationship between dentist and dying from uterine cancer is positive! The more people in a state who said that they visited the dentist, the more people (women) died of uterine cancer.

How can we interpret this result which is nothing short of bizarre? The first explanation is that it could not possibly be true. The statistical test suggests, however, that this finding is solid. The Sig value is .000 and its "t" value is sufficiently large at close to 4.

We know, however, that going to the dentist is linked with higher income and education so I checked the model to see if the dentist result may lose out when in competition with socioeconomic correlates. I will do this again to be certain. I confirm again now that the dentist item survives the challenge from my items for income, education, percent Black, Hispanic, Asian, and Jewish. Apparently, it is not a replacement for socioeconomic and ethnicity items because it survives these tests.

Why might going to the dentist result in a higher death rate from uterine cancer? The only thing I can think of is dental x rays. Dentists or others might have a better explanation for this enigmatic finding.

Repeating the procedure for this second uterine cancer model, we can use the equation numbers from the B column in the middle box of Table 13-8 to construct a "best view" of the pattern of uterine cancer by minimizing the sizeable effect of older age. Like before, we substitute the average value for percent age 65 but use the actual state values for the other two items.

For those unfamiliar with the way the numbers are presented for air pollution and dentist, we simply move the decimal two places to the left for a more conventional form which we can do when we write the equation.

Using the B column in the middle box of Table 13-8, we can now create this "best view" predicted death rate list. -3.699 + (.244 * 12.653) + (.08791 * pmmetro) + (.04806 * dentlvis). Following the instructions inherent in the above equation, the SPSS 11 statistical software package does the calculations for us, thankfully, putting in the appropriate values for each state for the two items we wish to vary, air pollution and dentist, while holding constant the effect of age by plugging in the average value for all the states instead.

The result is the "best view" list of predicted death rates from uterine cancer in Table 13-9. This list is largely the result of air pollution being linked with more deaths and visiting the dentist also being linked with more deaths (surprisingly).

The list in Table 13-9 shows that the lowest predicted death rate is in Wyoming and the highest is in Michigan. Because air pollution is still in this second model and has a large effect, the northeast states as well as California do not do well. They find themselves toward the bottom of this list of predicted deaths from uterine cancer, meaning a higher predicted death rate in those states.

Table 13-9 [uterdenl] uterine dentist list.

An alternative best view predicted death rate listing for uterine cancer based on actual deaths between 2012 and 2014. This model uses going to the dentist (more deaths!) instead of ultraviolet (fewer deaths). Once again, we push aside the effect of older age (more deaths) in order to gain a clearer view of the other two items: particle air pollution (more deaths) and visiting the dentist (more deaths)!

Wyoming	2.96	South Carolina	3.76
Oklahoma	3.06	New Hampshire	3.80
North Dakota	3.11	Alabama	3.81
Montana	3.13	North Carolina	3.82
Nevada	3.17	Nebraska	3.83
Idaho	3.25	Minnesota	3.95
Louisiana	3.27	Utah	3.97
Alaska	3.32	Tennessee	3.99
Mississippi	3.35	Indiana	4.02
West Virginia	3.36	Georgia	4.05
Arkansas	3.38	Massachusetts	4.12
New Mexico	3.41	Wisconsin	4.13
Kentucky	3.49	Ohio	4.14
South Dakota	3.52	Delaware	4.15
Florida	3.52	Rhode Island	4.15
Oregon	3.56	Pennsylvania	4.18
Missouri	3.58	New York	4.20
Washing	3.59	District	4.24
Kansas	3.59	Illinois	4.26
Hawaii	3.60	Maryland	4.32
Texas	3.65	Virginia	4.33
Colorado	3.65	New Jersey	4.33
Arizona	3.69	California	4.65
Vermont	3.72	Connecticut	4.68
Iowa	3.73	Michigan	4.82
Maine	3.73		

Having now presented both alternative models for dying from uterine cancer, which is better? Is it related to not strong enough ultraviolet as suggested in the first model or to visiting the dentist (too often?) as suggested in the second model. To a large extent, they are equal equivalent models and hence, possibilities.

I should note that, even I, priding myself on being open to new explanations, am hard pressed to accept the reasonableness of the finding that going to the dentist might increase the risk of dying from uterine cancer. This reluctance on my part flies in the face of the testing here which seems to suggest that the result is valid. I presented this second model for fear that there could be some uterine cancer danger from the dentist.

My overall preference, however, is for the first model suggesting that dying from uterine cancer is perhaps linked with insufficient exposure to ultraviolet in sunlight that is strong enough. As a final point, It IS interesting to note that particle air pollution (more deaths) is an item that appears in both models.

Chapter 14. Cervical Cancer Linked with NOT Visiting the Dentist (and Keeping One's Teeth Clean Enough) as well as with African Americans

For cervical cancer, we begin with Table 14-1, the death rate from cervical cancer by state in 2014-2016 per hundred thousand people, (including women and men). This state level death rate goes from about one death per hundred thousand to 3 deaths. Of course, among women only, the rate is about double.

For this cancer, there are four states with missing data, really that there were so few deaths (under 10, I believe) that government researchers considered the number too small to construct a reliable death "rate". From the original 51 cases (the states plus the capital city of Washington, District of Columbia), that leaves us with 47, still over the minimum number of 30 needed to do statistical analysis.

Thankfully, this problem of missing cases, while not desirable, proved not to be a stumbling block. The sizeable Adjusted R Square for the model as a whole in Table 14-5, top box, of .804, means that the model explains over 80 percent of the pattern between states in deaths from this cancer.

Looking more closely at Table 14-1, the lowest death rate from cervical cancer is for Utah (.9, less than one death per hundred thousand) and the highest is for Mississippi (2.8 deaths).

There are three items linked with death rates from cervical cancer. The first is visiting the dentist (Table 14-2) linked with FEWER deaths from this cancer. The second item is African Americans (percent black in 2005 [black05]) linked with more deaths (Table 14-3). The third item is age 65 and over [age65in6] linked, of course, with more deaths as well (Table 14-4).

In size order, the first is visiting the dentist over the past year, found in Table 14-2. West Virginia has the lowest percent of the population that visited the dentist over the past year, about 53 percent. Connecticut has the highest percent at about 79 percent. The higher the percent of the population in a state that visited the dentist over the past year, the lower the death rate from cervical cancer in that state.

Percent African American by state can be found in Table 14-3. These numbers are likely from census data based on self identification as belonging to one of a list of groups.

Table 14-1 cer1214a cervical 2012-2014

Death rate from cervical cancer by state in 2012 to 2014 per hundred thousand population including women and men. Four states are missing because they were designated "unreliable" because there were too few deaths from this disease.

State	Rate	State	Rate
North Dakota	.	Nebraska	1.6
Alaska	.	New Jersey	1.6
Vermont	.	California	1.6
Rhode Island	.	Nevada	1.7
Utah	.9	Indiana	1.7
Massachusetts	.9	Pennsylvania	1.7
New Hampshire	1.1	Wyoming	1.8
Minnesota	1.1	Georgia	1.8
Wisconsin	1.1	Illinois	1.8
Idaho	1.2	Texas	1.9
Washington	1.2	South Carolina	1.9
Colorado	1.2	Ohio	1.9
Oregon	1.3	New York	1.9
Hawaii	1.3	Kentucky	2.0
Virginia	1.3	Missouri	2.0
Connecticut	1.3	Tennessee	2.0
South Dakota	1.4	Delaware	2.0
Kansas	1.4	Louisiana	2.1
Maine	1.4	Oklahoma	2.2
Iowa	1.5	Florida	2.2
Maryland	1.5	District	2.2
Michigan	1.5	West Virginia	2.3
Montana	1.6	Arkansas	2.4
New Mexico	1.6	Alabama	2.6
Arizona	1.6	Mississippi	2.8
North Carolina	1.6		

Table 14-2 [dentlvis] dental visits. Percent in a state who visited the dentist over the past year.

State	%	State	%
West Virginia	53.1	Arizona	68.9
Mississippi	57.1	California	69.0
Oklahoma	57.8	Colorado	69.2
Arkansas	58.5	Oregon	70.2
Louisiana	58.9	Pennsylvania	70.2
Nevada	59.2	Illinois	70.6
Alabama	60.1	Iowa	70.8
Kentucky	60.2	Alaska	71.1
Missouri	60.8	Delaware	71.1
Texas	61.7	New York	71.2
North Dakota	62.9	District	71.4
New Mexico	64.2	Vermont	71.7
Montana	64.3	Maryland	71.9
Georgia	64.7	Nebraska	72.4
Wyoming	65.4	Utah	72.9
Idaho	65.7	New Hampshire	72.9
Indiana	66.6	Minnesota	72.9
Ohio	66.6	Virginia	73.1
South Dakota	66.9	New Jersey	73.6
Kansas	67.0	Rhode Island	75.4
South Carolina	67.0	Wisconsin	75.5
North Carolina	67.1	Massachusetts	75.9
Maine	67.2	Hawaii	77.0
Tennessee	67.5	Michigan	78.0
Washington	67.9	Connecticut	79.1
Florida	68.8		

Table 14-3 [black05] blacks.

Percent of the state population that identifies as black (African American) in 2005. (Montana is .43 percent black, or less than a half of one percent).

State	Value	State	Value
Montana	.0043	Kentucky	.0750
Idaho	.0056	Nevada	.0774
Vermont	.0064	Oklahoma	.0775
Maine	.0076	Indiana	.0885
South Dakota	.0077	Connecticut	.1009
North Dakota	.0078	Pennsylvania	.1060
Wyoming	.0079	Missouri	.1150
Utah	.0097	Texas	.1169
New Hampshire	.0099	Ohio	.1193
Oregon	.0181	Michigan	.1434
Iowa	.0233	New Jersey	.1448
Hawaii	.0235	Illinois	.1511
New Mexico	.0244	Arkansas	.1573
West Virginia	.0319	Florida	.1573
Washington	.0353	Tennessee	.1682
Alaska	.0361	New York	.1738
Arizona	.0364	Virginia	.1989
Colorado	.0409	Delaware	.2062
Minnesota	.0425	North Carolina	.2176
Nebraska	.0432	Alabama	.2639
Kansas	.0590	South Carolina	.2926
Wisconsin	.0598	Maryland	.2929
Rhode Island	.0613	Georgia	.2976
California	.0674	Louisiana	.3309
Massachusetts	.0686	Mississippi	.3694
		District	.5699

Table 14-4 Older Age. Percent of the state population that is age 65 and Over in 2006.

State	%	State	%
Alaska	6.8	Kentucky	12.8
Utah	8.8	New Jersey	12.9
Georgia	9.8	Kansas	12.9
Texas	9.9	Oregon	12.9
Colorado	10.0	Wisconsin	13.0
California	10.8	New York	13.1
Nevada	11.1	Oklahoma	13.2
Idaho	11.5	Nebraska	13.3
Washington	11.5	Massachusetts	13.3
Virginia	11.6	Vermont	13.3
Maryland	11.6	Missouri	13.3
Illinois	12.0	Connecticut	13.4
Minnesota	12.1	Delaware	13.4
Wyoming	12.2	Alabama	13.4
North Carolina	12.2	Ohio	13.4
Louisiana	12.2	Montana	13.8
District	12.3	Rhode Island	13.9
New Mexico	12.4	Arkansas	13.9
New Hampshire	12.4	Hawaii	14.0
Indiana	12.4	South Dakota	14.2
Mississippi	12.4	North Dakota	14.6
Michigan	12.5	Iowa	14.6
Tennessee	12.7	Maine	14.6
Arizona	12.8	Pennsylvania	15.2
South Carolina	12.8	West Virginia	15.3
		Florida	16.8

Percent black in 2005 goes from a low of less than a half percent (.0043) in Montana to a high of about 37 percent in Mississippi (second highest). The highest percent in Washington DC, counted in this analysis as a state but more like a city-type state, is about 57 percent (.5699) self-identified as black. The higher the percent black in a state, the higher the death rate from cervical cancer in that state.

The third and final item is age 65, the percent of the population in the state that are senior citizens, age 65 and over, found in Table 14-4. Alaska has the fewest seniors as a percent of the population. "Young" states include ones at the top of that list such as Utah, Texas, Colorado, California and Nevada. "Old" states are at the bottom of the list including Rhode Island with about 14 percent seniors, Hawaii similar, Pennsylvania around 15 percent, West Virginia a little higher and the highest state being Florida with close to 17 percent of the population in this older age category in 2006. As expected, the higher the percent age 65 and over, the higher the death rate from cervical cancer.

Now that we are familiar with the components, we can turn to the model itself for cervical cancer in Table 14-5. As is our pattern, we start with the bottom box to check that there are no large correlations between the items in the model. We do note a negative association between visiting the dentist and percent black (-.127). The more blacks in a state, the fewer people have been to the dentist. This association is quite small in size still, and is not designated statistically significant with one or two stars. The size of the other numbers are even smaller. All in all, this is a clean model fulfilling the assumptions of the method of the items being largely "uncorrelated".

While down in the bottom box, we note the bottom row showing the "zero order" correlations between each item and the matter at hand, death rates from cervical cancer by state during the years 2012-2014. These are only of passing interest because the combined model tells us more pertinent information about the effect of each item on cervical cancer after already accounting for the effect of the other items (to be more certain that each effect is "independent").

Nevertheless, we do see a sizeable connection between going to the dentist and cervical cancer (-.688**). The direction of this relationship is "negative". This means that the more people who have been to the dentist, the fewer deaths there are (per hundred thousand people) from cervical cancer.

Table 14-5 The Cervical Cancer Model:
The role of visiting the dentist (fewer deaths).

Model Summary

Model	R	R Square	Adjusted R Square	Std. Error of the Estimate
1	.904[a]	.817	.804	.1903

a. Predictors: (Constant), AGE65IN6, DENTLVIS, BLACK05

Coefficients[a]

Model		Unstandardized Coefficients		Standardized Coefficients	t	Sig.
		B	Std. Error	Beta		
1	(Constant)	3.285	.421		7.802	.000
	DENTLVIS	-4.465E-02	.005	-.615	-9.346	.000
	BLACK05	1.940	.241	.532	8.054	.000
	AGE65IN6	9.295E-02	.019	.318	4.843	.000

a. Dependent Variable: CER1214A

Correlations

		DENTLVIS	BLACK05	AGE65IN6	CER1214A
DENTLVIS	Pearson Correlation	1	-.127	-.065	-.688**
	Sig. (2-tailed)	.	.374	.6	000
	N	51	51	51	47
BLACK05	Pearson Correlation	-.127	1	-.075	.570**
	Sig. (2-tailed)	.374	.	.602	.000
	N	51	51	51	47
AGE65IN6	Pearson Correlation	-.065	-.075	1	.284
	Sig. (2-tailed)	.653	.602	.	.053
	N	51	51	51	47
CER1214A	Pearson Correlation	-.688**	.570**	.284	1
	Sig. (2-tailed)	.000	.000	.053	.
	N	47	47	47	47

**. Correlation is significant at the 0.01 level (2-tailed).

The simple connection with percent black is also large and solid at (+).570**. The higher the percent black in a state, the higher the death rate from cervical cancer. Older age, the final number, is not significantly linked (no stars) with cervical cancer in these direct relationships. This means that, only after accounting for the other items, the link with older age becomes apparent.

Next we move to the top box to look at the model's Adjusted R Square of .804. The model as a whole explains the pattern of differences in death rates across the states to a large extent, accounting for over 80 percent of the pattern.

Finally now, we are ready for the middle box in Table 14-5, the actual model. Glancing first at the right Sig. column, we see that all items have the value .000, the best. This is based on the numbers in the next column to the left "t" which need to be 2 or greater. These numbers are all large. Starting with the last of older age, the value is 4.8, suggesting the connection between older age and dying from cervical cancer is a solid one.

The other items have even larger numbers. The link between percent black and dying from cervical cancer in the "t" column has a value of 8, even more solid. Finally, the top item, visiting the dentist over the past year, has a value of 9 (leaving aside the minus sign right now), the highest of all. This means the connection in this model that we have uncovered between visiting the dentist and (fewer deaths from) cervical cancer is extremely solid based on this statistical test.

Next we move to the middle Beta column in the middle box of Table 14-5. I use this column to view the size of each effect relative to the other because the size of each number (ignoring the decimal and the sign for now) can be directly compared to the others.

We start by paying attention to the direction of the effects. The first, dentist, is negative while the other two have no signs which means positive (an imaginary +). The negative one means more people visiting the dentist, FEWER deaths. Turning that around, fewer people visiting the dentist, more deaths from cervical cancer. Positive means, more blacks, more deaths. Age 65 is also positive meaning more older people, more deaths.

Now we look at the size of the numbers. The items are arranged in size order. First, if all these items represent one hundred percent (of the explained portion of the pattern), how much out of that total is each item? To figure this out, we add up the three numbers together (ignoring the signs and the decimals) to reach a total and divide each by that total. (615+532+318=1465).

Dentist [dentlvis] is 615/1465=.4198 or 42 percent of the total. Percent black [black05] is 532/1465=.363 or 36.3 percent of the total. Older age [age65in6] is 318/1465=.217 or 21.7 percent of the total.

More interesting, however, is how big an effect each item is of the total POSSIBLE explanation of the pattern between states (of dying from cervical cancer). These numbers will be smaller because the model explains only some 80 percent of the total explanation. 1465/[80.4 (Adjusted R Square as a percent)]=x/100. 80.4x=146500. x=146500/80.4. x=1822, the larger number we can now use as the new denominator.

As a portion of the total possible explanation, dentist is 615/1822=.3375 or 33.8 percent of the complete explanation. Percent black is 532/1822=.292 or 29.2 percent of the total explanation. Older age is 318/1822=.1745 or 17.5 percent of the total explanation, both the part captured by this model and the part not captured by it.

Perhaps a few comments are in order about these results. Starting with the smallest effect of the three, older age, it is well known that older age is typically linked with dying in general as well as with dying from cancer. Apparently, this is also the case for this kind of cancer, cervical cancer (among women, of course).

What does it mean that percent African American is linked with explaining a sizeable part of the variation in death rates between states. We know that this connection is positive in direction. The most likely explanation of this result is that more African Americans die of it. There could well be a concentration of deaths in this group. While other possibilities exist for this finding, this straightforward conclusion seems the most plausible. It is my impression that this link between African Americans and cervical cancer is well known.

In my eyes, the most interesting result is the connection with going to the dentist. The direction of this connection is negative. The higher the portion of the population that has been to the dentist over the past year, the lower the death rate from cervical cancer. This connection is both very solid and quite large in size accounting for a full third (33.8 percent) of the pattern of differences between states in dying from this cancer.

When trying to understand this finding, what first comes to mind is the possibility that this connection must be misspecified. Perhaps the most reasonable explanation has nothing to do specifically with the dentist. Rather is must be due to the characteristics of the kinds of people who happen not to go to the dentist. We can assume that going to the dentist is a socioeconomic indicator of higher income, education or perhaps ethnic background none of which are specifically related to the dentist itself.

To test this reasonable alternative possibility, I will now use the final model but this time, include other items as a test: income, education, and some measures of ethnicity, such as Hispanics, Asians, and Jews. I will also add as further tests wine drinking (an indicator of higher socioeconomic status, perhaps surprisingly) as well as reading the newspaper every day. None of these "tests" threatened the final model, (not a surprise because I likely tested these things while developing the final model). "Dentist" easily survived these additional challenges.

The alternative idea for the dentist result as an indicator of higher socioeconomic status fails this rigorous test. We are, thus, left with the original idea that there is something specific about going to the dentist that is, itself, linked with fewer death from cervical cancer.

What might this effect be of going to the dentist? Two bacterial threats are dental caries (cavities) in teeth and periodontal disease in the gums. A leading few strains of bacteria in the mouth have been identified as centrally linked with each problem. Actions taken by the dentist might reduce problems leading to such disease.

In my broader interpretation of visiting the dentist, I make the assumption that people who have visited the dentist might be more motivated to care for their teeth and gums through "oral home care", flossing and brushing among other behaviors. To me, this large and solid connection between visiting the dentist and fewer deaths from cervical cancer suggests that there could be a hitherto unknown connection between dangerous mouth bacteria and the development of cervical cancer in woman leading to death.

Finally, we can construct a better view of death rates from cervical cancer by state for the years 2014, 2015 and 2016 from Table 14-1, one that is more illuminating. While it is an easy decision to hold constant older age, thus minimizing its impact, it is more difficult to decide how to handle the connection between cervical cancer and the size of the African American portion of the population. It makes the most sense, overall, while keeping in mind this strong connection with African Americans, to reduce its impact on the result by holding this item constant as well. This allows us to have a clearer look at the impact of the interesting "behavioral" item of visiting the dentist.

Using the left most "B" column in the middle box of Table 14-5, we can use this main summary of the model in numerical form, this equation, to accomplish the goals we decided on above. We can dramatically reduce the impact of the two demographic items (age 65 and percent black) by using the all-state averages. For our item of greatest interest, the dentist, we use the actual state values from Table 14-2. Of course, the original equation is influenced by these other two items so they do play a role regardless - despite the fact that this "best view" minimizes that role.

The all-state average for age 65 is 12.653 percent. (Typically, considering all the states together, a little under 13 percent of the population are in the senior age group). The all-state average for percent black in 2005 is .112761 or around 11.3 percent. (Today, it is probably about 13 percent but we use the specific number from the item that worked in the model). The two unfamiliar ways of noting the numbers can be changed by moving the decimal point two spaces to the left which we can now do in the following equation. 3.285 - (.04465 * dentlvis) + (1.940 * .112761) + (.09295 * 12.653).

This equation yields the "best view" list in Table 14-6. This is the predicted death rate from cervical cancer per hundred thousand (women and men) based on actual deaths between 2012 and 2014. As the only item to vary is "visiting the dentist", the ordering of the states is the same as on the list [dentlvis] in Table 14-2 but in the opposite direction. (This is due to the fact that the connection is negative, fewer who visited, more deaths). The second difference with the dentist list is that this new "best view" list includes a predicted rate for cervical cancer deaths for each state.

In this new Table 14-6, given that the prominent role is now about going to the dentist, Connecticut, the state with the highest proportion who see the dentist, has the LOWEST predicted death rate from cervical cancer. West Virginia, with the lowest percent of people who visit the dentist, has the highest predicted death rate from cervical cancer.

The list in Table 14-6 represents my best estimation of the most meaningful view of the pattern of cervical cancer deaths across the United States. This is after keeping in mind that the size of the black portion of the population in a state also affects actual rates as does the size of the senior citizen portion of the population.

Table 14-6 [cerdenl] cervical dental list.

Best view predicted death rate from cervical cancer by state per hundred thousand (women and men) based on actual deaths between 2012 and 2014. This view sets aside the effects of both older age (more deaths) and blacks (more deaths) in order to see more clearly the role of visiting the dentist (fewer deaths).

State	Rate	State	Rate
Connecticut	1.15	Washington	1.65
Michigan	1.20	Tennessee	1.67
Hawaii	1.24	Maine	1.68
Massachusetts	1.29	North Carolina	1.68
Wisconsin	1.31	Kansas	1.69
Rhode Island	1.31	South Carolina	1.69
New Jersey	1.39	South Dakota	1.69
Virginia	1.42	Indiana	1.71
Utah	1.42	Ohio	1.71
New Hampshire	1.42	Idaho	1.75
Minnesota	1.42	Wyoming	1.76
Nebraska	1.45	Georgia	1.79
Maryland	1.47	Montana	1.81
Vermont	1.48	New Mexico	1.81
District	1.49	North Dakota	1.87
New York	1.50	Texas	1.92
Alaska	1.51	Missouri	1.97
Delaware	1.51	Kentucky	1.99
Iowa	1.52	Alabama	2.00
Illinois	1.53	Nevada	2.04
Oregon	1.55	Louisiana	2.05
Pennsylvania	1.55	Arkansas	2.07
Colorado	1.59	Oklahoma	2.10
California	1.60	Mississippi	2.13
Arizona	1.60	West Virginia	2.31
Florida	1.61		

Chapter 15. Stomach Cancer Linked with Being Short and separately, with being African American

We now turn to stomach cancer in Table 15-1. Death rates by state from stomach cancer in 2012-2014 per hundred thousand population. Looking at the list, it goes from a low of 2.5 deaths in Utah to a high of 7.6 deaths in Hawaii.

As is our routine here, it is useful to first become somewhat familiar with the items used to explain the pattern of deaths from this cancer. There are two items linked with the pattern of stomach cancer deaths in the model and we can see these in the following two tables.

The first is height. Table 15-2 shows the average height of women in a state, the height item most strongly connected with stomach cancer. The shorter the average woman is in a state, the more deaths from stomach cancer there are. In the state of Hawaii, the height of the average woman is 63.15 inches or a little over 5-3, five feet three inches. In Utah, the height of the average woman is the tallest of all the states, 64.79 inches or a little less than 5-5, five feet five inches.

The model also works with height for both men and women averaged together but the best result is with the average height of women in a state. Obviously, this difference in average height of about two inches seems small. Nevertheless, it is this difference in the average height of women across the United States that works best for explaining the pattern of deaths from stomach cancer.

The second item of two (in this short model) is percent African American. This appears in Table 15-3. The higher the percent of the population that is African American, the higher the death rate from stomach cancer. This is the percent of the population that identified themselves as African American in 2005. This goes from a low in Montana with less than a half percent black (the actual number is .0043). The high is for Washington DC, called "District" in this list which stands for District of Columbia, not actually a state but treated as such in this research. Here the percent black is about 57 percent, (or .5699).

The model for stomach cancer deaths across the states is in Table 15-4. We start with the bottom box for zero order correlations primarily to make sure that the two items are reasonably independent of each other. This is important in order to fulfill the requirements of the method as well as to avoid erroneous results.

Table 15-1 [stom1214] stomach 2012-2014.
Average annual death rate by state from stomach cancer between 2012 and 2014 per hundred thousand population.

State	Rate	State	Rate
Utah	2.5	North Carolina	4.3
Nebraska	2.5	Kentucky	4.4
Wyoming	3.0	Arkansas	4.4
Colorado	3.3	Michigan	4.5
Kansas	3.3	Tennessee	4.5
South Dakota	3.3	Pennsylvania	4.6
Idaho	3.3	Massachusetts	4.7
New Hampshire	3.4	Delaware	4.7
Iowa	3.4	Texas	4.7
North Dakota	3.4	Florida	4.8
Montana	3.5	Connecticut	5.0
Minnesota	3.6	Illinois	5.0
Maine	3.6	Alabama	5.1
Indiana	3.9	Alaska	5.2
Missouri	3.9	New Jersey	5.3
Nevada	3.9	West Virginia	5.3
Virginia	4.0	California	5.4
Oregon	4.0	Louisiana	5.4
Arizona	4.0	South Carolina	5.5
Oklahoma	4.0	New Mexico	5.5
Vermont	4.1	New York	5.7
Washing	4.1	Rhode Island	5.8
Wisconsin	4.2	Mississippi	6.0
Ohio	4.2	District	6.2
Georgia	4.2	Hawaii	7.6
Maryland	4.3		

Table 15-2 [hitinchf] height in inches female. Average height in inches among adult females in a state. (In Hawaii, the average height among women is a little over 5-3, (five feet, three inches).

State	Height	State	Height
Hawaii	63.14	Missouri	64.51
Rhode Island	63.94	Iowa	64.53
New Mexico	63.99	Mississippi	64.53
New Jersey	64.06	Colorado	64.55
Massachusetts	64.07	Arkansas	64.57
Pennsylvania	64.20	Oklahoma	64.57
California	64.20	Wisconsin	64.58
Florida	64.23	District	64.58
New York	64.23	South Carolina	64.59
Connecticut	64.24	Illinois	64.59
Texas	64.25	Delaware	64.60
Vermont	64.25	Georgia	64.60
Alaska	64.32	Tennessee	64.61
Maine	64.32	Idaho	64.62
West Virginia	64.34	Nevada	64.62
Kentucky	64.36	Alabama	64.64
Louisiana	64.38	Wyoming	64.66
Michigan	64.38	Arizona	64.67
North Dakota	64.44	Montana	64.67
Indiana	64.44	Washington	64.70
New Hampshire	64.46	South Dakota	64.72
Kansas	64.47	Oregon	64.73
Ohio	64.48	Nebraska	64.73
Virginia	64.48	Minnesota	64.74
Maryland	64.49	Utah	64.79
North Carolina	64.51		

Table 15-3 [black05] black 2005.
Percent of the state population that identifies as black (African American) in 2005. The so called state with the largest percent black is District of Columbia - 56.99 percent or around 57 percent.

State	Value	State	Value
Montana	.0043	Nevada	.0774
Idaho	.0056	Oklahoma	.0775
Vermont	.0064	Indiana	.0885
Maine	.0076	Connecticut	.1009
South Dakota	.0077	Pennsylvania	.1060
North Dakota	.0078	Missouri	.1150
Wyoming	.0079	Texas	.1169
Utah	.0097	Ohio	.1193
New Hampshire	.0099	Michigan	.1434
Oregon	.0181	New Jersey	.1448
Iowa	.0233	Illinois	.1511
Hawaii	.0235	Arkansas	.1573
New Mexico	.0244	Florida	.1573
West Virginia	.0319	Tennessee	.1682
Washington	.0353	New York	.1738
Alaska	.0361	Virginia	.1989
Arizona	.0364	Delaware	.2062
Colorado	.0409	North Carolina	.2176
Minnesota	.0425	Alabama	.2639
Nebraska	.0432	South Carolina	.2926
Kansas	.0590	Maryland	.2929
Wisconsin	.0598	Georgia	.2976
Rhode Island	.0613	Louisiana	.3309
California	.0674	Mississippi	.3694
Massachusetts	.0686	District	.5699
Kentucky	.0750		

Table 15-4 The Stomach Cancer Model: the role of shorter height (more deaths).

Model Summary

Model	R	R Square	Adjusted R Square	Std. Error of the Estimate
1	.869[a]	.755	.744	.4999

a. Predictors: (Constant), BLACK05, HITINCHF

Coefficients[a]

Model		Unstandardized Coefficients		Standardized Coefficients	t	Sig.
		B	Std. Error	Beta		
1	(Constant)	172.290	16.592		10.384	.000
	HITINCHF	-2.614	.258	-.729	-10.147	.000
	BLACK05	4.718	.612	.554	7.708	.000

a. Dependent Variable: STOM1214

Correlations

		HITINCHF	BLACK05	STOM1214
HITINCHF	Pearson Correlation	1	.105	-.671**
	Sig. (2-tailed)	.	.465	.000
	N	51	51	51
BLACK05	Pearson Correlation	.105	1	.478**
	Sig. (2-tailed)	.465	.	.000
	N	51	51	51
STOM1214	Pearson Correlation	-.671**	.478**	1
	Sig. (2-tailed)	.000	.000	.
	N	51	51	51

**. Correlation is significant at the 0.01 level (2-tailed).

The correlation in this case is low in size at .105 and without stars meaning no significant connection at either the level of .05 or .01. Nice and clean.

We glance at the bottom row to see the direct correlations with the matter of interest, deaths from stomach cancer by state. Both are independently connected with stomach cancer, each with two stars, passing the more stringent statistical test at the .01 level. The correlation between the average height of woman in a state and death rates from stomach cancer in 2012-2014 is negative (-) .671. The negative sign means that the shorter the average woman, the more deaths from stomach cancer. For blacks, the connection is positive (no sign means a plus sign). The more blacks as a percent of the population, the higher the death rate from stomach cancer in that state.

Next we look at how well the model did in explaining the pattern across states by noting the Adjusted R Square in the top box of Table 15-4. It is .744, reasonably high, a good thing. This short model of two items explains 74.4 percent of the pattern, almost three quarters of the total possible.

The model itself appears in the middle box of Table 15-4. As always, we start with the level of significance which we use to have a rough idea of the solidness of these associations. The sig. value .000 is the best possible. The column one-to-the-left, labeled "t", shows that these numbers, which must be above 2, are actually way above. For the connection between blacks and stomach cancer, it is a little less than 8. For the link between (shorter) height and stomach cancer, t is over 10.

For the matter of interest, stomach cancer (as is the case for all of the other cancers as well), we can construct a meaning that we are dealing with a sample from a larger population. In point of fact, however, these death rates are, basically, a list from the death registry of ALL of the people in the United States who died of stomach cancer during this three year period. From these raw numbers, a yearly average is created and converted into a rate for each state. The numbers for blacks are probably from the US census from 2000 adjusted up for the additional extra five years. If so, this is no mere sample but is supposed to be an actual recording of deaths from this cause in the entire population.

Lastly, the height numbers, which I likely found in government statistics from a health survey, are highly accurate in my estimation even though it is based on self reporting. This is my first success with one of these lists for height being related to health matters.

We are now ready to view the actual model result, the first rendering being in the Beta (middle) column of the middle box in Table 15-4. The minus sign connotes more of one is linked with less of the other. The negative sign for height means that, as the average woman in a state is taller, there are fewer deaths from stomach cancer. The absence of a sign for blacks means a positive (+) sign is implied. The MORE blacks in a state as a percent of the population, the MORE deaths from stomach cancer (per population size).

These Beta numbers can be compared directly to each other in terms of size. First, we determine how big each items is in terms of one hundred percent. Obviously height is the effect that is larger in size. Ignoring the signs and the decimals, we now add the numbers together to determine the first denominator (729+554=1283).

For height [hitinchf], this is 729/1283=.568. This tells us that, of the portion of the pattern that the model explains, 56.8 percent of it is due to height, well over half. For the African American effect it is 554/1283=.432. Of the part that the model explains when trying to account for the pattern of differences between states in deaths from stomach cancer, the percent of the state population that is black explains 43.2 percent.

Overall, it is more interesting to know the absolute size of each effect as an explanation for stomach cancer death rates, both the majority part that the model succeeded to explain and the smaller part that the model failed to explain. Then we can talk more meaningfully about the role of each item as part of the full explanation. Of course, these numbers will be smaller.

To do this, we need the new larger denominator that represents the total explanation, the part explained by the model and the part not explained. Using the old denominator, 1283, as well as the Adjusted R Square, .744, we can figure this out. 1283/.744=x/1. 1283=.744x. x=1283/.744. x=1724.4623, the new denominator. Height is 729/1724.4623=.4227 or 42.3 percent of the total explanation. Percent black is 554/1724.4623=.321 or 32.1 percent of the total explanation. So in terms of the entire explanation for the pattern of deaths from stomach cancer, height among woman explains about 42 percent of the pattern while percent black explains a little less than a third of the pattern, about 32 percent.

What comments can I make about these results? Beginning with the smaller effect, as I stated earlier, if the percent of the population that is black is linked in a positive direction with the pattern of deaths from stomach cancer, the most reasonable explanation is that blacks themselves are more likely to die from this cancer. While highly likely, we actually cannot be certain that such is the case. It is still possible that a more esoteric explanation might be the truth. Perhaps the size of the black population might link with some other characteristic of the state in terms of lifestyle that has nothing directly to do with blacks. Here we will assume the more likely possibility stated above.

As for why blacks might be more likely to die of this cancer, I do not know. While blacks are categorized as a "racial" group, they are also a living social group that can be compared with many ethnic and language subgroups in the diverse population of the United States. Each has its own subset of distinctive cultural preferences on the one hand, while sharing in the country's common cultural norms on the other.

One possibility could be diet but, of course, this is only a guess and I do not know more specifically. Then there is the possibility of some inherited predisposition toward this kind of cancer. This would not be unusual because there are other examples of certain death patterns more common in certain parts of the population. Personally, I tend to downplay the role of physical inheritance and place an emphasis on lifestyle differences between groups as a more likely explanation. Unfortunately, there is nothing in the final model that can help us with this question of why African American are more likely to die from stomach cancer than the population as a whole, (if this is, indeed, the case which it probably is).

The second large effect is (shorter) height. The pattern of deaths from stomach cancer across the states in the US is linked with shorter height among woman. Height explains about 42 percent of the total pattern.

How can we best explain that it is height among woman rather than height in general, or among men, that best links to this pattern of cancer deaths? To repeat, the model also works with the average for height for women and for men combined. In my interpretation, I chose not to emphasize the "women" part and speak of it as a connection with height.

In general, I have no explanation for this height finding. I do not believe it to be a random fluke as statistical correlations are sometimes explained as being. While always a possibility, given the solid evidence from the statistical test (a t score higher than 10) as well as the hefty size of the effect, I believe we have to pay close attention to the possibility that such is the case, that for reasons unknown, shorter height is linked with dying from stomach cancer.

While I have no explanation for the result, it is vitally important to clarify that the best evidence suggests that the connection is with height specifically. Nevertheless, it is reasonable to consider the logical possibility that height differences between states might actually suggest groups of different ethnic and racial origin which might be shorter in height compared to the general population. If true, then height would "fall out" and be replaced with one or more such groups.

I thought of a way to test this alternative explanation. From various indirect statistical tests here, all on a state level, such groups with shorter average height may include Asians, Hispanics and Jews. Now I add these possibly shorter groups to the model to watch what happens. It is no contest. While the beta for height goes down to (-.625) in this preliminary model with the three group challenges, the Sig. value remains .000 and all three groups are clearly not statistically significant. While height is in the model, there is no significant connection between dying from stomach cancer and percent Asian, percent Hispanic or percent Jewish.

Before deciding finally that there is no connection between these origin groups (which might be shorter in height) and stomach cancer, we now redo the model without height. I will remove height now and replace it with these three groups. No connection with percent Jewish. No connection with percent Hispanic.

There is, however, a solid connection with percent Asian after removing height. In this alternative, but smaller, model, percent Asian sig .000, t value 5.9, beta .570, Adjusted R Square for this alternative model .532.

When I add height into this two-item alternative model, percent Asian drops out as it is no longer significant. Furthermore, the model Adjusted R Square jumps back up to .748 (before actually removing percent Asian from the model).

We learn from this alternative model, then, to my mild surprise, that there IS a connection between Asians and stomach cancer, larger in size, in fact, than the one with blacks. (Conventional spelling uses a capital letter for certain groups and a small letter for blacks for reasons unclear. By following the convention, I intend no slight).

The statistical significance of this connection is eliminated, however, once height is introduced. This teaches us that Asians as a group might be more prone to dying from stomach cancer but that this connection loses its distinctiveness, based on these statistical tests, once the more important and "genuine" explanation is introduced - shorter height.

This smaller and less important model suggested that being Asian might be linked with dying from stomach cancer. The bigger, better, final model corrects this conclusion, however. In the end, stomach cancer is not linked with being Asian per se but rather with being shorter in height.

Lastly, we want to use the actual equation for the final model with height and percent black to construct a "best view" version of the original list for stomach cancer deaths in Table 15-1. We can do this by using the numbers of the actual equation for the model which summarizes the model in numerical form to make a purposeful manipulation which should result in such a clearer view of deaths from this disease.

While the specific changes are a matter of judgment, the best path seems clear. Percent black is a standard demographic division of the population. The newest finding here is about shorter height and its connection with dying from stomach cancer. We can thus "hold constant" percent black (by using its all-state average) and in so doing, get a clearer view of the effect of shorter height on these death rates from stomach cancer.

The average percent black for the population across all the states happens to be a little more than 11 percent (.112761). We will now use the numbers in the B column of the middle box in Table 15-4 to write the equation allowing height to vary (by using the actual values for average height among women in the state from Table 15-5). For percent black [black05], we use the mean value (.112761).

The equation that can lead us to this "best view" predicted death rates from stomach cancer is as follows (from the B column in middle box in Table 15-4). 172.290 - (2.614 * hitinchf) + (4.718 * .112761).

We now instruct the SPSS 11 statistical software program to run this equation for each state. What results is the list in Table 15-5 Best view predicted death rate from stomach cancer per hundred thousand people.... As the only item that varies in this list is height, this ordering of states is the opposite of the height list in Table 15-2.

Because the association is "negative" with one going up, the other down, Utah in the record of average height in Table 15-2, with the tallest average woman, has the lowest predicted death rate from stomach cancer in Table 15-5. Also, Hawaii, with the shortest average woman, has the highest predicted death rate from this cancer in Table 15-5. The shorter the average height of women in a state, the greater the predicted death rate from stomach cancer.

Table 15-5 [stomhitl] stomach height list. Best view predicted death rate from stomach cancer per hundred thousand people based on actual death rates between 2012 and 2014. Here, the effect of the African American portion of the population is set aside (more deaths) in order to have a clearer view of the role of shorter height (more deaths). Please note that this ordering of states is the same as in Table 15-2 height female but the order is in reverse. This is because as average women's height goes down, stomach cancer deaths go up.

State	Rate	State	Rate
Utah	3.47	Maryland	4.24
Minnesota	3.60	Virginia	4.27
Nebraska	3.61	Ohio	4.27
Oregon	3.61	Kansas	4.28
South Dakota	3.65	New Hampshire	4.31
Washington	3.69	Indiana	4.38
Montana	3.76	North Dakota	4.39
Arizona	3.77	Michigan	4.54
Wyoming	3.81	Louisiana	4.54
Alabama	3.86	Kentucky	4.59
Nevada	3.90	West Virginia	4.64
Idaho	3.91	Maine	4.70
Tennessee	3.92	Alaska	4.70
Georgia	3.96	Vermont	4.87
Delaware	3.96	Texas	4.87
Illinois	3.99	Connecticut	4.89
South Carolina	4.00	New York	4.91
District	4.01	Florida	4.91
Wisconsin	4.02	California	5.00
Oklahoma	4.03	Pennsylvania	5.00
Arkansas	4.04	Massachusetts	5.33
Colorado	4.10	New Jersey	5.38
Mississippi	4.13	New Mexico	5.56
Iowa	4.15	Rhode Island	5.69
Missouri	4.20	Hawaii	7.76
North Carolina	4.20		

Chapter 16. Men Dying from Liver Cancer is Linked to Frequent Sexual Activity

Here, I refer to cancer of the liver and bile ducts simply as liver cancer. The model I choose to present is for men who died in 2013. These death rates are already adjusted for age so we are unable to assess the role that older age plays as a factor.

The original liver cancer death rate list can be found in Table 16-1. Our work is an attempt to explain the pattern of differences in these rates of death between states. Because these numbers have already been adjusted for age and are for men only, it is difficult to compare the size of this cancer with other kinds included in this study.

The lowest death rate is in Vermont with 5 deaths per hundred thousand and the highest is in Washington DC (District of Columbia) where the death rate is around 16 deaths. It is unclear to me whether the population size used to calculate the rate is for men only or for both genders.

As is our pattern, I introduce the items that come out in the model as helping to explain the pattern between the states of dying from liver cancer. There are three items linked with liver cancer in the final model in Table 16-5, the details of which will be examined a little later.

The first is the percent of the population in a state that is African American. The higher it is, the more deaths from liver cancer. It is highly likely that such is the case because blacks are more likely to die from liver cancer compared with the general population.

The second linked item is shorter height among men. This "height" connection is "negative" in direction meaning, the shorter the average height of men in a state, the more deaths from liver cancer. The reason for this connection with height is an enigma, most unclear.

The third connection is with frequent sexual activity. In a sex survey, when both men and woman were asked about frequency, one of the categories was "sex four times a week". The higher the percent of people in a state who gave that as their answer, the higher the death rate among men from liver cancer. As this result demonstrates a connection between frequent sex and dying from liver cancer, it raises the possibility that multiple partners might be involved but this is, of course, speculation.

Table 16-1 Death rate for Liver cancer (and bile duct) among men only in 2013, rate already adjusted for age

State	Rate	State	Rate
Vermont	5.0	New Hampshire	9.0
North Dakota	5.8	Florida	9.1
South Dakota	6.0	Georgia	9.1
Idaho	6.3	Arizona	9.3
Utah	6.4	Washington	9.3
Minnesota	7.2	Missouri	9.4
Nebraska	7.2	Oregon	9.4
Iowa	7.3	Tennessee	9.5
Wisconsin	7.3	New York	9.6
Montana	7.6	Maryland	9.7
Wyoming	7.6	Arkansas	9.9
Colorado	7.7	Delaware	10.1
Connecticut	7.7	North Carolina	10.1
Maine	7.9	Oklahoma	10.4
Kansas	8.1	Alaska	10.8
West Virginia	8.2	Massachusetts	10.9
Nevada	8.3	Alabama	11.2
Virginia	8.4	Mississippi	11.3
Michigan	8.5	California	11.5
New Jersey	8.5	Rhode Island	11.8
South Carolina	8.5	New Mexico	11.9
Ohio	8.6	Texas	11.9
Kentucky	8.7	Hawaii	12.5
Indiana	8.8	Louisiana	12.5
Pennsylvania	8.9	District	15.9
Illinois	9.0		

Table 16-2 [black05] black 2005.
Percent of the state population that identifies as black (African American) in 2005. The state with the smallest percent black is Montana -.43 percent or under a half percent.

State	Value	State	Value
Montana	.0043	Nevada	.0774
Idaho	.0056	Oklahoma	.0775
Vermont	.0064	Indiana	.0885
Maine	.0076	Connecticut	.1009
South Dakota	.0077	Pennsylvania	.1060
North Dakota	.0078	Missouri	.1150
Wyoming	.0079	Texas	.1169
Utah	.0097	Ohio	.1193
New Hampshire	.0099	Michigan	.1434
Oregon	.0181	New Jersey	.1448
Iowa	.0233	Illinois	.1511
Hawaii	.0235	Arkansas	.1573
New Mexico	.0244	Florida	.1573
West Virginia	.0319	Tennessee	.1682
Washington	.0353	New York	.1738
Alaska	.0361	Virginia	.1989
Arizona	.0364	Delaware	.2062
Colorado	.0409	North Carolina	.2176
Minnesota	.0425	Alabama	.2639
Nebraska	.0432	South Carolina	.2926
Kansas	.0590	Maryland	.2929
Wisconsin	.0598	Georgia	.2976
Rhode Island	.0613	Louisiana	.3309
California	.0674	Mississippi	.3694
Massachusetts	.0686	District	.5699
Kentucky	.0750		

These three connected items can be found in the following tables. Starting with Table 16-2, we have the percent of the population that identifies as African American in 2005. The lowest percent is in Montana where a little less than a half percent identify as black (.0043 or .43 percent). The highest "state" is Washington DC, considered here a state, at .5699 or about 57 percent black. The state with the second highest percent black is Mississippi, whose black population is 36.94 percent of the state population (or around 37 percent).

The average height among men in a state is in Table 16-3. The chart is in inches. In Hawaii, the state with the lowest average height among men, this is 68.30 inches or a little over 5-8, 5 feet 8 inches tall. The state where the average height of men is highest is Arkansas. There men average 70.70 inches in height or a little less than 5-11, (5 feet 11 inches). To repeat about direction, the lower the average man's height in a state, the more deaths from liver cancer.

The item about the frequency of sexual activity is in Table 16-4. This is the percent of people in a sex survey who, when asked how often they had sex, chose the reply "four times a week". (As best as I recall, this was the highest frequency choice). It goes from a low in Rhode Island of 4.7 percent who chose that option to a high in Arkansas where 7.5 percent chose the reply of "four times a week". To repeat about direction, the higher the percent of respondents to this sex survey who answered this "most frequent" reply, the more deaths in that state from liver cancer. I will comment about this later in greater detail.

Now that we are familiar with the items linked with liver cancer in the model, we are ready to examine the liver model itself in Table 16-5. As usual, we start in the bottom box with the correlations between the items. We note that this examination shows a problem-free lack of connectedness between the items. None of these correlations are statistically significant (neither one nor two stars) and the sizes of the correlations are small. This is a good thing, fulfilling the requirement of the regression method. It is also good in that it minimizes the possibility of one common cause of erroneous results which might lead us astray.

Finally, we glance at the bottom row of this bottom box in Table 16-5 to look at the connections between each item and the matter of interest here, dying from liver cancer in 2013. Already in these zero order correlations, all three items are linked with liver cancer with two stars, at the .01 level of significance.

Table 16-3 [hitinchm] height inches men. Average height among men in a state in inches (from a health survey).

State	Height	State	Height
Hawaii	68.30	Virginia	70.36
New York	69.64	Nebraska	70.39
New Mexico	69.65	Missouri	70.43
California	69.72	South Carolina	70.43
Rhode Island	69.84	West Virginia	70.43
New Jersey	69.87	Idaho	70.44
Texas	69.88	Kentucky	70.45
District	69.89	Alabama	70.45
Massachusetts	69.89	Kansas	70.46
Arizona	69.89	Iowa	70.46
Connecticut	69.90	Wisconsin	70.47
New Hampshire	69.98	North Carolina	70.48
Alaska	70.02	Indiana	70.48
Nevada	70.05	Oregon	70.52
Ohio	70.06	Colorado	70.52
Vermont	70.07	Washington	70.56
Florida	70.08	Wyoming	70.56
Maine	70.10	Tennessee	70.56
Louisiana	70.17	Minnesota	70.60
Oklahoma	70.18	Georgia	70.61
Pennsylvania	70.19	South Dakota	70.64
Maryland	70.21	Utah	70.66
Delaware	70.24	Montana	70.67
Michigan	70.26	Mississippi	70.67
Illinois	70.34	Arkansas	70.70
North Dakota	70.36		

Table 16-4 [psex4xpw] percent sex 4 times per week.
Percent who said they had sex four times a week
(in a sex survey).

Rhode Island	4.7		South Dakota	5.4
Massachusetts	4.7		New Mexico	5.6
Connecticut	4.7		Arizona	5.6
New Hampshire	4.7		Nevada	5.6
Vermont	4.7		Idaho	5.6
Maine	4.7		Colorado	5.6
Ohio	5.2		Wyoming	5.6
Michigan	5.2		Utah	5.6
Illinois	5.2		Montana	5.6
Wisconsin	5.2		New York	5.7
Indiana	5.2		New Jersey	5.7
District	5.3		Pennsylvania	5.7
Florida	5.3		Kentucky	6.4
Maryland	5.3		Alabama	6.4
Delaware	5.3		Tennessee	6.4
Virginia	5.3		Mississippi	6.4
South Carolina	5.3		Hawaii	7.2
West Virginia	5.3		California	7.2
North Carolina	5.3		Alaska	7.2
Georgia	5.3		Oregon	7.2
North Dakota	5.4		Washington	7.2
Nebraska	5.4		Texas	7.5
Missouri	5.4		Louisiana	7.5
Kansas	5.4		Oklahoma	7.5
Iowa	5.4		Arkansas	7.5
Minnesota	5.4			

Table 16-5 The Liver Cancer Model (men).
The role of shorter height (more deaths) and sex four times a week (more deaths).

Model Summary

Model	R	R Square	Adjusted R Square	Std. Error of the Estimate
1	.840[a]	.705	.686	1.1187

a. Predictors: (Constant), PSEX4XPW, BLACK05, HITINCHM

Coefficients[a]

Model		Unstandardized Coefficients		Standardized Coefficients	t	Sig.
		B	Std. Error	Beta		
1	(Constant)	164.248	27.837		5.900	.000
	BLACK05	10.066	1.366	.585	7.367	.000
	HITINCHM	-2.291	.395	-.463	-5.807	.000
	PSEX4XPW	.814	.189	.343	4.301	.000

a. Dependent Variable: LIVMEN13

Correlations

		BLACK05	HITINCHM	PSEX4XPW	LIVMEN13
BLACK05	Pearson Correlation	1	.045	.057	.584**
	Sig. (2-tailed)	.	.753	.691	.000
	N	51	51	51	51
HITINCHM	Pearson Correlation	.045	1	-.099	-.471**
	Sig. (2-tailed)	.753	.	.487	.000
	N	51	51	51	51
PSEX4XPW	Pearson Correlation	.057	-.099	1	.423**
	Sig. (2-tailed)	.691	.487	.	.002
	N	51	51	51	51
LIVMEN13	Pearson Correlation	.584**	-.471**	.423**	1
	Sig. (2-tailed)	.000	.000	.002	.
	N	51	51	51	51

**. Correlation is significant at the 0.01 level (2-tailed).

Between percent black and liver cancer in men, the correlation is (+).584**. More blacks, more deaths. Between men's height and liver cancer, the correlation is -.471**. Shorter height among men, more deaths from liver cancer among men. Lastly, the correlation between sex four times a week and men dying from liver cancer is (+).423**. The higher the percent of people saying they have sex this often, the more deaths from liver cancer among men.

Next, we can move to the top box in Table 16-5 to see the Adjusted R Square of .686. This model explains 68.6 percent of the pattern between states. I chose this particular model based on this score, slightly higher than numbers for liver cancer among both men and woman in the same year of 2013 as well as higher than an earlier model based on a list from between one and one and half decades ago.

Given that these numbers for liver cancer among men are already age adjusted, this result for the total explanatory power of the model is probably on the high side. This is because, typically, older age is a weighty item which contributes substantially to the size of the model's explanatory power in these attempts to explain the pattern of deaths from various cancers.

Finally, we move to the main part, the middle box in Table 16-5 with the actual final model. First we start with the right two boxes which test the statistical significance of the connections between each item and the subject of interest, liver cancer. I consider it important as an indicator of the solidness of the connection between each item and liver cancer.

Starting on the right, the Sig. column shows values of .000, the best. This is because the numbers in the next column "t" are so big. They should be over 2 but these are much larger. The connection between blacks and liver cancer is very solid with a t value over 7. The connection between shorter height in men and liver cancer has a t value of almost 6. The connection between frequent sex and liver cancer has a smaller value of 4 but still well over 2.

Moving to the left now, we reach the Beta column in the middle box of Table 16-5. These are listed in size order. The biggest in size of the three effects is blacks as these numbers can be compared in size to each other (after ignoring the signs). The implied sign is a plus (+) or positive. This means that the higher the percent black in a state, the more deaths among men in that state from liver cancer.

We cannot be certain that this means it is black men themselves who are more likely to die from this cancer. Nevertheless, this large and solid connection appears to imply that something powerful is linking these two items with each other. Just to mention another esoteric possibility, the percent black might represent some social characteristic of the population of the state that we have not thought of and it is that characteristic that would be related to dying from liver cancer. The most likely possibility, however, is the straightforward one, that black men are significantly more likely to die of liver cancer than the male population as a whole.

This next number is the Beta value for average height among men in a state -.463. This is the size (compared to the other numbers) of the connection with liver cancer. It has a minus sign for negative in direction. The lower the height of men, the more deaths from liver cancer among men.

Last is the percent who say they have sex four times a week. The Beta is (+).343. More people who have sex four time a week, more deaths among men from liver cancer.

We can now use these Beta numbers to make some assessment of the strength of each item (relative to the others) as a factor explaining deaths from liver cancer among men. First, we ask how big is each item as a portion of the explanation that the model succeeded in capturing. We know from the Adjusted R Squared, that this is 68.6 percent of the total possible. To do this, we ignore the signs (and the decimals), add the numbers together to get a denominator. Then we divide each Beta number by that denominator. 585+463+343=1391.

For blacks, it is 585/1391=.421 or 42.1 percent of the explanation we have uncovered here. For height, it is 463/1391=.333 or 33.3 percent of the explanation we have come up with here. Lastly, for sex four times, it is 343/1391=.245 or 24.5 percent of the part of the explanation we have here.

A still more meaningful description of size is what these results mean in terms of the total possible explanation of the pattern. The model succeeds in explaining 68.6 percent, a little over two thirds of the possible. What would be the size of each effect in terms of the total possible explanation?

We know that the previous denominator of 1391 represents 68.6 percent of the explanation so we can easily use this relationship to come up with a new, larger denominator which would represent one hundred percent, the entire explanation that is possible. 1391/.686=x/1. .686x=1391. x=1391/.686. x=2027.697, which is now our new denominator.

For blacks, it is 585/2027.697=.2885 or 28.9 percent of the total possible explanation. For men's height, it is 463/2027.697=.228 or 22.8 percent of the total possible explanation. For frequent sex, it is 343/2027.697=.169 or 16.9 percent of the total possible explanation.

The B column in the middle box of Table 16-5 contains the actual final equation which represents a numerical summary of the result. Before using this equation to create a new best look at the pattern, now might be a good time for some comments on the results so far.

In terms of the size of the effects, the most important thing to know, which helps determine the pattern of deaths from liver cancer among men, is the portion of the state population that happens to be African American. Knowing that one detail helps to explain 28.9 percent of the difference in dying between states or over a quarter. As already stated, this suggests, albeit indirectly, that men dying from liver cancer is, likely, concentrated, to a considerable extent, among blacks.

It seems that this pattern linking blacks to liver cancer has strengthened over the past decade. Any over-time analysis in this research is extremely rare. For this cancer, however, I have examined another model of deaths from liver cancer among both men and women from this disease from one to one and a half decades earlier (not shown). In that model, the effect linking blacks to liver cancer was last in size of the three and it is now first in size. As for what might explain this certain increased concentration, I do not know.

The next-in-size item to explain the pattern across the states of men dying from liver cancer is shorter men's height. This explains 22.8 percent of the pattern or a little over a fifth. The shorter men are in a state, the more deaths there are in that state from liver cancer among men.

Clearly, this result is difficult to explain. I am not entirely surprised by the finding in the sense that I always believed that these slight variations in average height, from a national government survey on self reported height, were high in quality. While men might exaggerate their height over the telephone, the key is that such exaggeration does not vary between states in a way that would ruin the relationship of each state number with the other states. Another way to say this is that, even though there might be some embellishment, it is not necessarily a problem as long as men in one state do not engage in it more than men in another state.

The interesting question here is why height might be related to dying from liver cancer. (While this model is for men, I should note that the same model works for all deaths from liver cancer including those among women, a model not shown). In light of its unexpected character, this relationship would be a good candidate for the alternative explanation that height itself, while technically strong, might not be the most meaningful connection to note. Rather, perhaps it was something else connected to height.

What comes to mind is certain "origin" groups (or ethnic groups) of the American population which might be shorter when compared to all Americans. I happened to come across indirect evidence that such might be the case using this particular measure for average height among men. There is a negative association with three origin groups including percent Asian (correlation between men's height in a state and percent Asians (-.757**), percent Hispanic (-.454**) and percent Jewish (-.403**). This is a correlation between the height of men and the percent of each group (which includes woman as well) in a state. Perhaps the genuine connection with liver cancer is not with height but rather with some or all of these groups.

The idea is easy to test by adding items for all of these groups into the model to see what happens. None of these group items are significantly connected with men dying from liver cancer. In fact, height is completely unchallenged by the test maintaining its Sig. score of .000, the best.

Apparently, then, it is not that these groups, whose men might be shorter, are related to dying from liver cancer but rather it is being shorter per se that is related. It is men's height, in the end, that is connected with liver cancer. The connection appears not to be specifically with any of these groups where people might be shorter than the general population.

Given the evidence here, it is my hunch that it probably IS height itself that is responsible for the finding. While I don't know specifically why height might relate to deaths from liver cancer among men, it could have something to do with the connection between height and one's location in the hierarchy of male society. Perhaps height has some effect on sexual behavior although I prefer not to go into more detail because the thinking is highly speculative broaching a subject about which human knowledge is probably limited.

The last of the three items related to dying from liver cancer (among men) is the frequency of having sex. The specific connection is between the percent of the sample representing the state's population who answered that they had sex four times a week. (More who say they have sex four times a week, more liver cancer deaths). This item about sex frequency explains 16.9 percent of the total pattern or a little less than a fifth of the entire possible explanation. While this is the smallest size result of the three, it seems clear to me that it is the most weighty in terms of its significance.

There is no clear indication in this item whether the sex four times a week is with the same or different partners. This general connection with sex raises the possibility, however, that, in relative terms, some of these might be people with multiple partners. Furthermore, we have no information about the kind of sexual contact involved.

From elsewhere, however, we know about the link between liver cancer and a sexual transmitted virus, Hepatitis C. One becomes infected through contact with an infected partner's bodily fluids including blood and semen with saliva less of a factor. I choose not to go into more detail here due to a lack of exact understanding about transmission and the various kinds of sexual contact that are most likely involved. Once infected with this typically sexually transmitted virus of Hepatitis C, after a delay in time, liver cancer can follow.

It is in this context of the important role of Hepatitis C in the development of liver cancer that we can best understand the main finding of this model. While perhaps this is largely known, the result in this research, showing a solid connection between frequent sexual activity and liver cancer, might be confirming statistical evidence, however imperfect in terms of the lack of details, pointing to the possible role of frequent sexual activity.

While this possibility stretches the actual result past what might be certain, it seems plausible to me that this indicator of frequent sex might represent sex with multiple partners engaging in "unprotected" sex which would entail exposure to Hepatitis C. This might, in turn, lead to the eventual development of liver cancer. While plausible, due to the limitations of the specific result, this possibility must remain in the realm of speculation.

Nevertheless, given what we know about the link between Hepatitis C and liver cancer, the result here appears to provide further evidence that is statistical in nature that liver cancer might be, at its heart, a sexually transmitted disease linked with a virus.

While I do not spend time in this research on null (non-confirming) findings, perhaps it is important to mention in this context that I have found no connection between men dying from liver cancer and two well known connections mentioned over the years. The first is the connection with drinking (alcohol).

I have many good measures for alcohol consumption, purchase, various kinds, heavy drinking and none of these works in the model in that they fail the test of statistical significance at the .01 level. While such a null finding cannot definitely prove that drinking is unrelated to getting liver cancer and dying from it, the fact that this known connection cannot be discerned statistically, does, in my mind, question its centrality in the liver cancer story.

The same is the case for smoking cigarettes. My item called "smoking every day", which works fine for lung cancer (not shown), is not related in this model to men dying from liver cancer.

I bring up these null results in the context of the link found with frequent sexual activity. For me, it highlights a possible shift that may be in order which focuses attention more clearly on the link between sexual activity specifically and liver cancer.

With that uncomfortable topic now behind us, we can turn to the actual numerical summary of the result in the B Column of the middle box of Table 15-5. We want to use these numbers to write an equation that will provide us with a better view of deaths from liver cancer among men across the states of the American union. This is a matter of personal judgment because it results in an altered view of the actual death rate for men in 2013 from the starting numbers in Table 16-1.

For this new view, I have decided to reduce the effect of the largest item, percent African American, as a way of gaining a clearer view of the impact of the other two items. I do this by holding percent black "constant" by using the average value for all of the states which happens to be .112761 or 11.3 percent.

Of the remaining two items, I, obviously, want to let frequent sex vary to see its effect more clearly. We do this by using the actual value in each state (Table 16-4) for the percent of people who say they have sex four times a week.

I have also decided to let vary the middle item of men's height on the hunch that there is something important going on between men's average height and liver cancer even though I am not sure what that is. Once again, I do this in the following equation by going to Table 16-3 and using the actual value for the average height among men for each state.

To summarize, then, in the following "best view", predicted death rate list, percent black is held constant (to minimize its effect in this new view) while height and frequent sex are both allowed to vary. We can now write the equation and let the statistical software package, SPSS 11, generate the result for each state. This will give us a predicted value for deaths from liver cancer among men which will be our "best view" look at the pattern.

Using the numbers in the B column, we can now write this final equation. 164.248 + (10.066 * .112761) - (2.291 * hitinchm) + (.814 * psex4xpw).

Running this equation yields the final list in Table 16-6, the best view predicted death rate from liver cancer among men.... This predicted rate is based on the actual rate in 2013 for liver cancer deaths among men. The lowest predicted death rate is now Georgia at 7.94 deaths per hundred thousand or around 8 deaths and the highest is for Hawaii with 14.77 deaths or about 15 deaths.

This is the view we get after reducing the large effect of the size of the African American portion of the population on the result. In this new view, we get a better look at the role of frequent sex and shorter height on the pattern of dying from liver cancer.

To end on a personal note, I knew nothing about this particular cancer before working on this chapter. Of course, the whole project is rather dark because it involves a certain archeological excavation of people who already died of cancer. For some reason, I find the information resulting from the work here on liver cancer to be unusually unpleasant to learn about.

Table 16-6 [livmenl] liver men list.

Best view predicted death rate from liver cancer among men in 2013 after already accounting for the connection with percent black (more deaths). This allows a better view of the remaining two connections: average height among men (shorter, more deaths) and percent (both genders) who say they have sex four times a week (more deaths).

Georgia	7.94		New Hampshire	8.88
South Dakota	7.94		Tennessee	8.94
Minnesota	8.04		Connecticut	9.07
Montana	8.04		Massachusetts	9.09
Utah	8.06		Ohio	9.12
Indiana	8.14		Florida	9.15
Wisconsin	8.17		Rhode Island	9.20
North Carolina	8.23		Alabama	9.20
Wyoming	8.29		Kentucky	9.20
West Virginia	8.33		Pennsylvania	9.21
Iowa	8.34		Nevada	9.45
South Carolina	8.35		Arkansas	9.52
Kansas	8.35		District	9.58
Colorado	8.37		Washington	9.60
Virginia	8.43		Oregon	9.68
Missouri	8.43		Arizona	9.82
Illinois	8.47		New Jersey	9.95
Nebraska	8.50		New Mexico	10.38
Idaho	8.57		New York	10.47
North Dakota	8.59		Oklahoma	10.70
Maine	8.61		Louisiana	10.73
Michigan	8.66		Alaska	10.84
Vermont	8.67		Texas	11.38
Mississippi	8.69		California	11.53
Delaware	8.78		Hawaii	14.77
Maryland	8.85			

Chapter 17. Summary of Cancer Models in Three Tables and Some Almost Final Thoughts

In this chapter, I present three summaries of the results. Table 17-1 is the bare bones summary of the model for each cancer.

Table 17-2 (placed many pages forward after the discussion of the first table) is an even shorter version including only one connected item for each cancer model, the one I consider to be the most interesting. This is the shortest summary of the results so far.

Table 17-3 flips the connections around the other way. Here, the results are grouped by the connected item. Perhaps this is the most interesting new look.

Starting with Table 17-1, perhaps I will go down the list and add some final thoughts about each kind of cancer hoping not to repeat myself too much from the main chapter on each cancer. It is a way of providing a quicker summary for readers who are looking for that. Of course, it lacks the full effect of the nuance.

Please recall that the model yields what the connections are for each cancer but does not automatically provide evidence for the "why" question - why is each item connected with a particular cancer. So often, the uncovered connection seems surprising and perplexing.

In my attempt here to explain a connection, when I do have a hunch, this should best be viewed under the category of speculation. As we are toward the end now, perhaps my style is a little less formal and slightly more personal in places.

Beginning the discussion of the summary results in Table 17-1, the first model, "all deaths from cancer", is one of the most interesting ones. Yes, cancer is related to older age, smoking. The "Jews" finding is a surprise. For this disease, it seems probable that Jews are less likely than the general population to die from cancer. In the first chapter, I have no idea why this might be. I doubt it relates to some inherited physical difference because we are all so alike physically. The irony of the finding is that perhaps most people I know who died of cancer were Jewish, testimony to the difficulty of generalizing from your own experiences.

By the end of the second chapter, however, I figure out that a good part of the reason why Jews are less likely to die from cancer (compared with the population as a whole) is that they are less likely to live in households with a dog. I have a little more to say on this when discussing the next model.

The connection with rain is interesting but very enigmatic. The more inches of rain, the more deaths from cancer in that state. This also comes out in the next model called "all deaths from cancer minus lung cancer" which is the "all deaths" cancer numbers subtracting the lung cancer deaths from them.

What might the rain finding suggest? In this case, while, of course, it could be something directly about rain, I suspect that rain serves as the best summary for something else.

Table 17-1 Summary of the final models for each cancer.

All models are attempts to explain the pattern of deaths from cancer between states. + means association in same direction, - means association in opposite direction.

All deaths from cancer
Older age [age65in6] + (more seniors, more deaths)
Smoking cigarettes [smokrs96] + (more smokers, more deaths)
Inches of rain in largest city during the year [rain2] + (more rain, more deaths)
Percent Jews in a state [pjews96] – (FEWER Jews, more deaths)

All deaths from cancer minus lung cancer
Older age [age65in6] + (more seniors, more deaths)
Strength of Earth's magnetic field on the ground [geomag08] + [stronger magnetic field (roughly more north), more deaths]
Inches of rain in largest city during the year [rain2] + (more rain, more deaths)
Percent of households with a dog [doghouse] + (more such households, more deaths)

Lung cancer
College [sumcolig] – (more who attended college, fewer deaths)
Ultraviolet [uvi0614] – (stronger the ultraviolet reaching ground, fewer deaths)

Breast cancer (some 99 percent of deaths are among women)
Particle air pollution [pm07] + (more air pollution, more deaths)
Older age [age65in6] + (more seniors, more deaths)

Colon cancer
Older age [age65in6] + (more seniors, more deaths)
Visited the dentist [dentlvis] – (FEWER who visited the dentist, more deaths)
Smoking cigarettes [smokrs97] + (more smokers, more deaths)

Melanoma skin cancer
Percent of households with a dog [doghouse] + (more such households, more deaths)
Older age [age65in6] + (more seniors, more deaths)
Strength of ultraviolet in sunlight reaching the ground [ultra96] – (WEAKER ultraviolet, more deaths)

Urinary tract cancer (includes bladder)
Older age [age65in6] + (more seniors, more deaths)
Strength of ultraviolet in sunlight reaching the ground (at midday) between 2006- 2014) [uvi0614] - (WEAKER ultraviolet, more deaths)

Non Hodgkins lymphoma
Older age [age65in6] + (more seniors, more deaths)
Strength of Earth's magnetic field at location of largest city [magnetic] + [stronger magnetic field (roughly, more north), more deaths]

Pancreatic cancer (based on numbers for women)
Average altitude in the state [altstate] − (LOWER elevation, more deaths)
Consumption of wine during the year [ethpcwyn] + (more wine drinking, more deaths)

Adult Leukemia
Older age [age65in6] + (more seniors, more deaths)
Strength of Earth's magnetic field on the ground [geomag15] + [stronger magnetic field (roughly, more north), more deaths]
Percent of households with a dog [doghouse] + (more such households, more deaths)

Prostate cancer (men)
Older age [age65in6] + (more seniors, more deaths)
Strength of magnetic field on the ground in the largest city [magnetic] + [stronger magnetic field (roughly, more north), more deaths]

Ovarian cancer (women)
Older age [age65in6] + (more seniors, more deaths)
Strength of ultraviolet in sunlight reaching the ground [ultra96] − (WEAKER ultraviolet, more deaths)

Uterine cancer model 1 (women)
Older age [age65in6] + (more seniors, more deaths)
Particle air pollution in downtown of largest city over the year [pmmetro] + (more air pollution, more deaths)
Strength of ultraviolet in sunlight reaching the ground [ultra96] − (WEAKER ultraviolet, more deaths)

Uterine cancer model 2 (women)
Older age [age65in6] + (more seniors, more deaths)
Particle air pollution in downtown of largest city over the year [pmmetro] + (more air pollution, more deaths)
Visited the dentist [dentlvis] + (MORE who visited the dentist, more deaths!)

Cervical cancer (women)
Visited the dentist [dentlvis] − (FEWER who visited the dentist, more deaths)
Percent African Americans in a state [black05] + (more blacks, more deaths)
Older age [age65in6] + (more seniors, more deaths)

Stomach cancer

Height among women [hitinchf] – (SHORTER height, more deaths)
Percent African Americans in a state [black05] + (more blacks, more deaths)

Liver cancer among men

Percent African Americans in a state [black05] + (more blacks, more deaths)
Average height among men in a state [hitinchm] – (SHORTER height, more deaths)
Percent who say they have sex four times a week + (more who say four times, more deaths)

While just a guess, I suspect, after years of work on this related topic, that rain is linked with elevated gamma radiation probably from thunderstorms. On the other hand, the elevated gamma radiation could be in the rain itself picking it up from higher in the atmosphere. Rain might bring it along on the way down to the ground. It is only relatively recently that we have learned there is a "terrestrial" (Earth origin) source of gamma radiation. Gamma, of course, is the highest intensity range of the electromagnetic radiation spectrum.

Another possible version of this idea that "rain is really elevated radiation" is this. The posited elevated level of gamma radiation comes up from the ground during rain, or due to rain. Radiation is well known to be linked with cancer. Over the years, I have brought together measures for testing including ground radiation in different cities as well cosmic radiation.

The most useful item has been something called geomagnetic cutoff rigidity. Greater rigidity confers better protection from space radiation by keeping the lower energy portion of radioactive particles in the cosmic ray stream from entering the atmosphere. Consequently, they cannot reach the ground in places where the rigidity is high. Rigidity is another "north south" item as it is strongest (confers the best protection) at the equator and goes down in size as we move north toward the magnetic pole.

Despite my best hopes for showing some connection between naturally occurring radiation and cancer, it was to no avail. The simpler and more mundane item of "inches of rain over the course of the year" works better as an explanation for how many people die from cancer (after controls). (More rain, more cancer).

Maybe the rain result is actually some other weather item that is higher when there is rain. One example is moisture in the air. I have measures for that such as humidity and dew point but the model comes out rain, inches of rain.

In the end, I have not given up on the radiation explanation for the rain finding even though I am unable to prove it directly. Gamma radiation goes up the more rain there is and this must be why more people die from cancer. In truth, however, it remains an open question why rain is linked with cancer.

Moving to "all deaths from cancer minus lung cancer", it was my own idea to make a model for this cancer combination. To repeat from the main text, lung cancer is a substantial portion of all deaths from cancer (about 28 percent). For this reason, lung cancer might be large enough for any of its distinctive features to affect our understanding of cancer in general.

This turned out to be the case with smoking, at least to some extent. Indeed, without lung cancer, smoking is no longer an item explaining deaths from cancer. This can be confirmed by looking over the items in the second model in Table 17-1.

To my surprise, however, after years of being familiar with this, I learned in more recent models that smoking is linked with not only all deaths from cancer and lung cancer (even though it is not does not appear in the model presented earlier) but also with colon cancer.

In this look at all cancers without lung, we see first that rain still makes it into the model as related. This confirms its place of importance in my eyes.

The finding about having a dog (more cancer deaths) breaks my heart to mention. While I have never lived with a dog as a child or as an adult, I am well aware how precious pets are to their owners. Hating to mention this as well, I happened to come across a correlation between having a dog and lower income.

My hope was that the connection between dog and cancer was not real - that cancer, if from having a dog, is, instead, because of the true link it is expressing - between lower income and cancer. Alas, it does not appear to be the case when I checked out this alternative idea. If having a dog is related to cancer, I do not know what the mechanism might be that would bear responsibility for this connection.

At the end of this discussion about dogs and cancer with the exception of lung cancer in the original chapter, Chapter 2, I happened to come across a negative association between the percent of the state population that is Jewish and the percent of households in that state that have a dog. There is reason to suspect that Jews are less likely to have a dog. I conclude from additional testing that this could be a large part of the explanation for why it appears that Jews are less likely (than the entire population) to die from cancer. I further conclude that the Jews finding in the first chapter indirectly provides additional evidence for this connection between having a dog and cancer.

Finally, in this model for "all deaths minus lung", the big finding appears to link cancers with living "north", specifically the increasing strength of the Earth's magnetic field as we drive north. We can't feel it, of course, but this research suggests from several possibilities, that it is this increased strength of the magnetic field on the ground.

This field is not directly measured but, rather, estimated for each location using an Earth science model based on the physical attributes of the location, in this case, the largest city of the state. From the best science evidence I have been able to assemble, the link between living more north and dying from cancer, which seems very strong, might be due to these changes in the planet's magnetic field.

While I am uncertain about whether or not this connection might be reflected in "reality", the result here suggests that it is among the strongest possibilities that I have been able to uncover. If, in the future, additional evidence helps to confirm this link between too strong Earth magnetism and dying from cancer (minus lung), I have no clear idea to explain it.

In an added final chapter, I take a new look at cancer minus lung from Chapter 2. This simpler, alternative model confirms the northern pattern but presents a different explanation for it.

The next cancer in Table 17-1 is the largest individual cancer category, "lung cancer". Among more than one option, I chose to present the model with two items. Going to college is linked with fewer deaths while stronger ultraviolet in sunlight is also connected with fewer deaths.

As I brought up in the original chapter, college is linked with both older age (more seniors, fewer in the state who attended college) as well as with smoking (more who smoke every day, fewer who have attended college). Choosing college to be in the model made it impossible to have these other items in the model because it would create technical problems.

The link between lung cancer and insufficient ultraviolet reaching the ground in sunlight is the main result for this model. This connection is revealed through the use of an updated measure of ultraviolet. The UV Index from NOAA combines nine years of predicted ultraviolet reaching the ground when the sun is highest in the sky, around noon, when the ultraviolet portion in sunlight is strongest. This number for the largest city in the state is used to represent the state.

After accounting for the tremendous impact of college on state death rates for lung cancer, the final model reveals a solid effect of the size of the UV Index on the pattern of death rates for lung cancer from state to state. The more north we go (in the United States located in the Northern hemisphere, of course), the sun gets weaker. This includes its small ultraviolet portion.

While sunlight is radiation that is part of the electromagnetic spectrum, this spectrum is somewhat arbitrarily divided up into parts based on the frequency of the wavelength. Sunlight is often described as having three such parts including the largest part which is heat or infrared radiation. We can feel this but cannot see it. The second largest part is visible light. The smallest part, but the one with the highest energy, is ultraviolet, around five percent of the total. Humans are unable to see this part either.

As the ultraviolet keeps getting weaker (when we travel north), more people die from lung cancer. Surely, the uncovering of this connection, if correct, represents a notable result because lung is the largest cancer. More people die from it than any other cancer.

The "breast cancer" result, I feel, is striking. My mother's mother died of it around age 46 in the late 1930s, well before I was born. May the poor woman rest in peace. My mother loved her very much, gone now as well.

Breast cancer is related to air pollution. It is related to a particular kind of air pollution called particle pollution or particulate matter. To repeat, it is small pieces of dirt in the air made of carbon from car and truck exhaust as well as from power plants and factories. Now on the internet, we have real time posting of levels in different cities called airnow.gov.

What is distinctive about the research here is its macro nature showing a connection between air pollution and breast cancer across the entire country as a whole (using state death rates). While they probably were not able to measure air pollution as well during the 1930s, when my mother's mother died, it was likely present in the Brooklyn, New York of that time. Perhaps this helps to explain why this disease cut short her life.

While we have known that air pollution harms the lungs, there has been ever broadening research to suggest the damage goes further, and it is implicated in heart disease as well. The research here broadens the effect even further to cancer - by linking air pollution in a statistical model across the entire country with dying from one of the largest cancers, breast cancer. (Particle pollution is also linked with uterine cancer to be discussed further on).

The next cancer in Table 17-1 is colon cancer. According to the model, this cancer is linked with two things which are surprising to me. The first is smoking cigarettes.

Most readers would not be surprised because, for decades, "everybody" has known that smoking causes cancer. Then, I do this research and find that yes, smoking is related to lung cancer (model not shown) and yes, to all deaths from cancer too. However, when you remove lung cancer, the connection between smoking and other cancers (taken together) disappears. This is why I was surprised to find that it is back again as a factor with another particular kind of cancer, dying from colon cancer.

As for why such is the case, my guess is that the bacteria in the mouth and "gut" affect each other and that smoking alters the bacterial biome in the mouth.

More interesting still is the connection between not going to the dentist and dying from colon cancer. The interventions that dentists perform might well have an independent effect on health. These include the removal and filling of cavities (dental caries) as well as the removal of plaque through scaling and cleaning of the gums and teeth.

I tend to emphasize, however, the indirect meaning of visiting the dentist. Visiting may be a window into a regimen of daily oral care at home. Those who do not see the dentist may be less likely to keep current with a home regimen of flossing and brushing or whatever variations might be practiced. (As a personal example, I learned about the Waterpik Water Flosser Ultra Model from my dentist and I believe it has greatly contributed to my oral health).

Once again here, the mouth is connected with the stomach. It is quite likely that mouth bacteria, including unhealthy types, might overpopulate as a result of neglected daily oral care. They might then migrate to the gut and influence the bacterial profile there. This, in turn, might precipitate colon cancer and death from the same.

Elsewhere, there is evidence for the effect of mouth bacteria on heart disease with a certain bacterium related to gum disease (P. gingivalis) showing up in arterial plaque. This connection might be because the mouth is also connected, through respiration, with the lungs. Such bad mouth bacteria could end up, via the lungs, entering the bloodstream and circulating to far off parts of the body. This path is even less circuitous for the gut and the digestive system because food so easily connects the mouth and the gut. It is no surprise, then, that the bacterial biome of one might affect the other region as well.

Of course, the macro nature of this connection between not visiting the dentist and dying from colon cancer leaves the specific mechanism far from certain. Nevertheless, the finding here suggests that it might be fruitful to take a closer look at the possible connection between oral health and colon health.

The "melanoma skin cancer" finding might, overall, be one of the biggest surprises of the research. First, the link with having a dog is very likely new and might prove useful, if substantiated in other ways. As melanoma is a cancer of the skin, I would think that physical contact between the dog and human skin might be some sort of mechanism to explore. Exactly how and why such contact might result in cancer, I do not know.

To repeat, while I have never had a dog either as a child or an adult, I am well aware of the strong emotional bond of families with their dog and feel sad to bring up this topic. I only do so in the hope that the information might prove helpful.

While I happen to choose "having a dog" as the most interesting connection for melanoma in Table 17-2, perhaps the most explosive finding is the link between the sun's ultraviolet and dying from melanoma. After decades of believing that melanoma skin cancer is from exposure to the ultraviolet portion of sunlight, I come up with research here suggesting the exact opposite, that melanoma might, indeed, be linked with ultraviolet but in the opposite direction.

Dying from melanoma appears to be linked in some way to insufficient exposure to the sun and its ultraviolet, most likely to a sunlight whose ultraviolet is not strong enough.

I make the point by demonstrating that there are more deaths from melanoma, the more north we drive in the United States. This contrary pattern is best explained by the weakening of the ultraviolet in sunlight as we drive north.

The key to developing evidence for this novel result is a never before used (to my knowledge) "operationalization" (putting into number form) the strength of ultraviolet by employing a version of the UV Index (UVI) for each major US city. In the version used here, the extended time frame of a full year is used, the average value of strength of ultraviolet reaching the ground in a city.

As best as I know, this data was created especially for this research with the help of the kind NOAA scientist Craig Long, (done a second time as well over the extended time frame of this project in an update). Of course, he had no idea about the actual result in advance and cannot be held responsible for it in any way.

Equipped with this new way of representing the strength of ultraviolet in sunlight, I was able to show a connection in the model between weaker ultraviolet (as we move north) and more deaths from melanoma.

Of course, this way of measuring ultraviolet, a breakthrough on its own, is far from perfect in that it makes no attempt to measure exposure to this part of sunlight directly. This very macro state-level analysis, encompasses the entire known list of people who died from melanoma during the given three year period. It also includes the ultraviolet values for the largest cities across the entire United States. A smaller, more micro, study might have been able to come up with a way to measure the actual exposure of people to sunlight. In this grand look at the connection between ultraviolet and dying from melanoma here, such was not possible.

Through interpretation, there are perhaps ways of reconciling this result with conventional notions that retain the idea that melanoma is the result of skin burning from exposure to the ultraviolet portion in sunlight. Doing so, however, is not recommended given the contortions that are necessary to bring about such peace between the conventional explanation and this new renegade result.

To state the conclusion with even greater bluntness, if there are more deaths from melanoma as you drive north in the United States, as the sun and its ultraviolet portion become weaker and weaker, it seems unlikely that melanoma could be from strong ultraviolet.

I chose to present this ultraviolet model as the best one for melanoma because it was the most technically strong choice, despite the controversy I knew would result. With people's lives at stake, this was no time to play politics.

There are other possibilities as well for a connection with environmental items that vary with latitude. What seems difficult to challenge, however, is the general result making clear that, when driving from the south to the north in the United States, there are more deaths from melanoma along the way (after controls).

Perhaps some additional words are appropriate about the meaning of this controversial finding which more explicitly evaluate alternative interpretations. First, there is the possibility that, despite the clear result showing a link between less ultraviolet and more deaths from melanoma, perhaps this indirectly highlights other related possibilities.

One is that sunlight might still be the culprit and that this ultraviolet-weakened sunlight in more northern locations might accentuate skin burning from the infrared portion of sunlight – thus leading to melanoma. Actually, for years, I have been a believer in this idea that "filtered" sunlight, with the ultraviolet portion diminished, is dangerous. This would be the case with any filtering of ultraviolet, through car glass, through sunscreen creams, or through later-in-the-day sunlight when the ultraviolet portion is already greatly diminished.

While I have no intention of changing my personal behavior of avoiding such ultraviolet-diminished sunlight, the analysis in the melanoma chapter persuaded me that the notion is likely wrong. This is because, to the best that my numbers are able to discern with various tests, there is a high correlation between the three different portions of sunlight: infrared (heat), visible light and ultraviolet. When we drive north, if the strength of ultraviolet goes down, the strength of the other portions of sunlight go down as well, get weaker.

If it is a problem to argue that melanoma is from ultraviolet that gets weaker and weaker as we drive north, the same problem persists when arguing that it is from other parts of sunlight. To argue that melanoma is from infrared radiation in sunlight makes just as little sense because this portion too gets weaker and weaker as we drive north and more people die from melanoma.

Another option is to argue that melanoma could not possibly be from diminished ultraviolet. If there were ever a result that cries out for an alternative explanation, this is it. As is always possible, while the result shows a link between weaker ultraviolet and more deaths from melanoma, perhaps the genuine connection is between melanoma and something closely related to ultraviolet in its pattern of variation between places.

There are two strong candidates for such related, yet entirely different, items. The first is geomagnetism which varies strongly with ultraviolet even though in the opposite direction. As we drive north, while ultraviolet gets weaker, geomagnetism gets stronger. Maybe the real culprit for melanoma is Earth magnetism instead. While it is possible to build a reasonable model with magnetism instead of ultraviolet, I chose as the final model the one with ultraviolet because it was technically stronger.

The second possible alternative is radiation coming down from the sky as part of the stream of radioactive particles in cosmic rays. I have various ways to measure the strength of such a radioactive stream which, to a large extent, varies with altitude, the intensity being stronger at higher elevations. There is no connection, generally speaking, between deaths from melanoma and the strength of that cosmic ray stream.

There is a second feature of the cosmic radiation stream that does vary with latitude and therefore, seems to present a more promising alternative because ultraviolet as well varies as you drive north. A portion of the cosmic ray stream is affected to the ability of the planet's magnetic field to act as a shield against lower energy radioactive particles coming from the galaxy. Called geomagnetic cutoff rigidity, this shield works better at the equator but less well toward the magnetic poles where it allows into the atmosphere more such particles.

For this reason, more radioactive particles are able to reach the ground at higher latitudes (as a generalization). Because geomagnetic cutoff rigidity weakens as we drive north in the United States, then perhaps the real connection is between melanoma and not ultraviolet but rather more of these radioactive particles coming down from the sky as we continue driving north.

I tested these different measures connected to the idea of cosmic radiation, and, unfortunately or not, there is no connection that can be discerned using these statistical methods between such radioactive particles and melanoma. So once again with this alternative, we are left with the unusual result with which we started, a link between weakened ultraviolet and dying from melanoma.

There is one more substantive problem involved with causing resistance to the result as stated, that there is a link between weakened ultraviolet and deaths from melanoma. Of course, a big problem is political, in that the finding appears to dramatically weaken the consensus view that ultraviolet causes melanoma. There is nothing more I can say about that.

I do wish to mention one last problem – something about the nature of the finding itself. This main explanation for melanoma is a negative association. The less strong that ultraviolet is, the more deaths from melanoma. In a way, a negative association is inherently difficult to interpret.

Even here, I have done the best that I can in trying to understand this connection but it still remains inexact and a little confusing. In some places, I argue that perhaps it is the lack of exposure to sunlight and its ultraviolet portion that is involved with cells turning cancerous. Elsewhere, I express skepticism that differences in exposure to sunlight in different places seem a likely explanation for variations in the pattern of deaths as we drive north. Here I move to the idea of the weakening strength of the sun's ultraviolet itself. Perhaps it is too weak to "do the job" as we end up north enough on our hypothetical road trip – and that is the best explanation for why more people die of melanoma the more north we are.

Despite the difficulty caused by the fact that this association is negative in direction, I have decided that I can accept that feature of the result. While a little more difficult to interpret and understand, there is nothing technically inferior about a connection that is negative in nature, with one going down (ultraviolet) and one going up (melanoma). It is simply the way the result came out.

As an final important disclaimer, this finding linking dying from melanoma with sun that is insufficiently strong has nothing to say about skin cancer of other types, typically treated by dermatologists without resulting in death. I have been unable to find numbers for the incidence of such cancers that are national in scope. For this reason, one has to be careful in applying the conclusions here to this non melanoma skin cancer. It is my own belief that the research here has nothing to say about this topic.

Cancer of the urinary tract including bladder cancer is another cancer related to ultraviolet. The geographic pattern must be similar. As we drive from south to north, in the West, from San Diego to Seattle, in the East from Key West Florida, to Maine (on I-95 North), there are more deaths from bladder and other cancers of the urinary tract. Using a new updated measure for ultraviolet reaching the ground in major US cities during 2006-2014, I found a connection between the two, ultraviolet and cancer of the urinary tract. After accounting for older age, the connection appeared.

The weaker the ultraviolet reaching the ground around noon time, the more people die from urinary tract cancer. Once again, the particular result suggests that such cancer may be due, at least in part, to insufficient exposure to ultraviolet that is sufficiently strong.

Non-Hodgkin's lymphoma is another cancer with a south to north pattern and there are more deaths as you drive north. This time, however, the connection is with another environmental factor that varies so closely with latitude. As we drive north, the strength of the Earth's magnetic field increases. This field is also known as geomagnetism.

The result here suggests that it is this stronger Earth magnetism that is involved, most closely related to the increasing pattern of deaths the more north we go. How such increases in Earth magnetism might perhaps precipitate the development of Non-Hodgkin's lymphoma and death from the same, I do not know.

Pancreatic cancer is next on the list in Table 17-1. I very much wanted to include it because I have known several people over the course of my lifetime to die from it, including my uncle and my professor who was the head of my dissertation committee in graduate school, both of blessed memory.

Unfortunately, I had to go to a different set of numbers where death rates were organized by gender. I ended up using the list for pancreatic cancer deaths among women. That I recall, building a successful model for this particular cancer proved to be a challenge.

Given this unusual circumstance of developing a model for a cancer that kills both women and men based on numbers for one gender only, I cannot say whether the same applies for men as well. I include the numbers for men but for unknown reasons, it was far more difficult to develop a successful model from those numbers. My best guess is that the model explaining pancreatic cancer deaths for woman would apply for all deaths from this disease.

The final results are interesting but the second saddens me in particular. First, elevation or altitude, two words for the same thing as best as I understand, appears to be involved in the pattern of death from pancreatic cancer. This is an unusual finding and only one other cancer has an elevation component, lung cancer, which ends up not making it into the final model. The directions for these two cancers is the same with lower elevation being related to more deaths. The actual pattern of elevation is affected by the particular topography of the United States. There are mountain areas near the East and West coasts but the big elevation is in the area of the Rocky Mountains (in the western portion of the country).

Then there is the matter of the distribution of the population with the bulk of the population living in the lower elevation areas nearer the older settled part of the country in the East. Furthermore, in the United States, the lowest-down possibility is sea level, the level of the surrounding oceans.

Despite the uneven distribution of the population across various levels of elevation, the pattern for this cancer links dying from pancreatic cancer with the lower elevations [in a linear (straight line) relationship]. The lower down, the more deaths from pancreatic cancer.

Of note is the elevation items that works best to explain this pattern. This happens to be the average elevation of the entire state. Regardless, the general pattern that results with pancreatic cancer is that the lower down people live, the more deaths from this cancer.

Of course, the air becomes "thicker" at low elevation, more dense, meaning a greater availability of oxygen for breathing in the volume of air in front of the mouth and nose. Air is typically more moist as well, and also typically filled with more air pollution.

I did check different variations of such items. The result of these tests is that there is no significant connection between them and pancreatic cancer but the connection is confirmed between lower elevation and this cancer. Ultimately, however, I do not have a good idea about what feature of lower elevation explains how it might be linked with more deaths.

Pancreatic cancer is linked with a second item as well - drinking wine. In great contrast with food, I have found many kinds of alcohol measures on a state level including different kinds of alcohol - "spirits" (or hard liquor), beer and wine. Another measure is for binge drinking - heavy drinking on one occasion - about five drinks.

As for drinking and cancer, I have found no link in this research with one exception. This is in contrast with other research, one study finding a link between drinking and breast cancer. Here, I have not found evidence for such a connection that is large enough to show up in these macro level statistical models.

Of course, the entire finding is unfortunate because I do not like to learn that activities which give people pleasure are bad for health. This is all the more the case with wine after studies over the decades have found a benefit for wine drinking against heart disease. While it does not exactly surprise me, it does make me feel sad.

I do not know what might explain this connection between wine and cancer of the pancreas. One idea that occurs to me relates to the slight radioactivity of wine. Perhaps it is this feature of wine which helps to explain this connection. Wine is also slightly magnetic based on my own tests.

For adult leukemia, as I read down the summary list in Table 17-1, there is a connection between this cancer and having a dog (on the level of US states). More households with a dog in a state, more deaths in that state from adult leukemia. I don't know why.

The bigger finding is the connection between leukemia and a higher strength of Earth magnetism. This is based on a USGS estimate for the strength of geomagnetism in the largest city of the state using an online calculator. I do not know why stronger geomagnetism might be linked with more deaths from adult leukemia.

Next is "prostate cancer" (among men, of course). This cancer is also linked with the strength of the Earth's magnetic field. Stronger size of the magnetic field on the ground in that location (roughly, the more north you drive), the more deaths from prostate cancer. I do not know why.

The model for death rates from ovarian cancer (in women) by state comes out as also related to more deaths as you travel north. For this cancer, the connection appears to be clearly with ultraviolet. As you drive north, (in the hypothetical east coast example, from Key West Florida, to Bar Harbor, Maine, (two places to which I have driven), deaths from ovarian cancer increase. The model highlights the best explanation as the gradually diminishing intensity of sunlight along the way, specifically its tanning component called ultraviolet. As the ultraviolet gets weaker along the route, the death rate from ovarian cancer goes up.

In general, the research here compares people in different places (states) with each other. It does a poor job in explaining why some women in the same place get this cancer and die of it while others do not.

I think the best explanation for this result has to do with differences in the intensity of sunlight itself. If that intensity of sunlight (and its ultraviolet component) weakens as you drive north, then even what they call "incidental" exposure to sunlight might not help. While the broad research here is not capable of measuring "exposure" directly, if the sun is too weak to start with, it might not work to have its posited therapeutic value against this cancer (ovarian).

I wish to summarize my thinking in this final attempt for improved clarity. In one additional detail about my understanding, there are, of course, two components which might help to explain this finding linking weakened ultraviolet in sunlight with more deaths from ovarian cancer. While it is probably true that exposure of the skin to the sunlight must be necessary, it is hard to believe that such exposure might vary in a systematic fashion between places based on how north the place happens to be.

If so, then it must be the variation in the strength of the sunlight itself, its ultraviolet, that makes the difference. For women living too far north, even those who are out in the sun at the right time of day, around noon, might be at risk because the sunlight itself is not strong enough.

Of course, not only is it the time of day that plays a role but also the season of the year because sunlight is, of course, so much weaker in the winter.

For deaths from uterine cancer, there are several interesting connections. Perhaps the most striking is air pollution. Like with breast cancer, the death rate among women from uterine cancer is linked with particle air pollution, a well-followed and documented kind of air pollution consisting of tiny particles of dirt (carbon) so small that we cannot see them. The dirtier the air in the largest city of the state, the more women there are who die from uterine cancer in that state. This air pollution item shows up in both models for uterine cancer.

The two models diverge on the third item. In the first model, it is ultraviolet that is linked with uterine cancer, once again, a lack thereof. As you drive north, the sun gets weaker together with its ultraviolet portion and this weakening in strength is linked with more deaths from uterine cancer.

In the second variation, ultraviolet is replaced with a different item, the dentist. To my great surprise, visiting the dentist is linked with more deaths from uterine cancer. The only idea I can think of for explaining this unexpected finding (if correct) is dental x rays which might cause damage even though the two parts of the body are not particularly close to each other.

For cervical cancer, once again, there is a link with "dentist" but for this cancer, the connection is back to being in the expected direction. Not visiting the dentist is linked with a higher death rate from cervical cancer.

Once again, I presume this is the case because bad mouth bacteria might be breathed in and enter the blood stream through the lungs to end up affecting the cervix negatively, somehow leading to cancer.

The remaining two cancers are linked with an unusual item, height, and, more specifically, being shorter. For stomach cancer, the best connection is specifically with average height in a state among women. This height items is based on a telephone sample of respondents in that state during a health survey. The shorter the average woman in a state, the more deaths from stomach cancer. I do not know why.

The liver cancer model is for deaths among men, the numbers which worked best for constructing a successful model. Once again here, shorter height, this time among men, was linked with more deaths from liver cancer.

The most interesting result for liver cancer, however, was a link with sexual activity. This connection with sexual activity is specifically with having sex four times a week. Sex four times a week was connected with more deaths among men from liver cancer. I speculate here that the selection of this choice of four times a week might be an indication of multiple partners. This might provide indirect evidence for the known connection between the acquisition of the sexually transmitted virus of Hepatitis C and liver cancer.

While the interpretation of a connection with shorter height is enigmatic, I speculate vaguely that men's height might influence sexual activity due to its ancient association with the pecking order in male society.

Concluding the cancer models listed in Table 17-1, I do wish to note an important omission. In this brief summary, I have not discussed two demographic items, the ways people are different from each other. The first is the connection between different cancers and older age. The second is a connection between certain cancers and African Americans. I discuss both in the main text.

Table 17-2 is a shorter version of the summary in Table 17-1 that I just briefly described. Listing only what I consider to be the one most interesting connection, it is much shorter compared to the full listing in Table 17-1. While less complete, it might provide a quicker summary of the main results in the cancer models and perhaps a shorter review of the results from the above text.

I should note that, for this list, I chose having a dog as the most interesting connection for melanoma whereas in the longer text, I seemed to imply that the connection with ultraviolet was more interesting due to the contrarian character of that finding. I chose dog in Table 17-2 because the finding was so unexpected and is probably unknown until now.

Table 17-2 The one most interesting connection for each cancer

All death from cancer – rain (more rain, more deaths)

All deaths from cancer minus lung cancer - Earth magnetism (stronger, more deaths)

Lung cancer – ultraviolet (less intense ultraviolet in sunlight, more deaths)

Breast cancer – particle air pollution (more pollution, more deaths)

Colon cancer – dentist [fewer who visit (insufficient oral hygiene?), more deaths]

Melanoma skin cancer – dog (more households with a dog, more deaths)

Urinary tract cancer including bladder – ultraviolet (weaker ultraviolet, more deaths)

Non-Hodgkins lymphoma – Earth magnetism [stronger (more north), more deaths]

Pancreatic cancer (among women) – wine (more wine, more deaths)

Adult Leukemia – dog (more households with a dog, more deaths)

Prostate cancer – Earth magnetism [stronger (more north), more deaths]

Ovarian cancer – ultraviolet (weaker ultraviolet, more deaths)

Uterine cancer – particle air pollution (more air pollution, more deaths)

Cervical cancer – dentist [fewer who visit (insufficient oral hygiene), more deaths]

Stomach cancer (among women) – height (shorter, more deaths)

Liver cancer (among men) – frequent sex (more who say four times a week, more deaths)

Lastly is a final and different kind of summary in Table 17-3 Cancer results groups by connected item. This turns the results around from describing specific cancers to grouping cancers according to specific items. This way, for the first time, we can see more clearly which cancers have connected items in common. This is my favorite summary of the project so far. The table first lists 11 items connected with the different cancers. Then, another four items are the characteristics of people in the various states (demographic in nature) that are related to deaths from cancer.

In the following summary, bad means more deaths and good means fewer deaths. The eleven connected items, following along from Table 17-3, are as follows: 1. Earth magnetism (bad), 2. Ultraviolet (good), 3. Dentist (mostly good), 4. Dog (bad), 5. Smoking (bad), 6. Air pollution (bad), 7. Rain (bad), 8. Wine (bad), 9. Height (taller good), 10. Frequent sex (bad) and 11. Elevation (good).

The four demographic items linked in these models with cancer are number 12. College (fewer deaths), 13. Blacks (more deaths), 14. Jews (fewer deaths) and 15. Seniors (more deaths).

Below these items, the particular cancers that are linked to each are listed together.

What have we learned about cancer from this project? Perhaps Table 17-3 - grouped by connected items - provides the best summary for answering this question. A large number of cancers are related to "living north" compared to places that are less north. This could be from the stronger magnetism of the planet itself as we move farther north (in the United States) and away from the equator. It might also be the weaker sun, most likely its tanning part, ultraviolet, as we move farther from the equator where the sun is strongest.

Insufficient oral hygiene seems to be centrally connected with cancer, two kinds, as the connection with whether or not we have seen the dentist. In my own interpretation, diligent daily care of the teeth at home is important for preventing certain cancers. Strangely, for one cancer, uterine, death rates are higher in states where more people have visited the dentist.

Having a dog seems to be linked with different cancers, to my chagrin.

While no surprise, smoking is linked with two cancers, colon, and lung, (indirectly in the selected model through its strong connection with not attending college). The connection with colon cancer was surprising to me. Due to the huge size of lung cancer among all cancers, smoking is also linked with all deaths from cancer.

Table 17-3 Cancer Results Grouped by Connected Item

These connections were determined in individual models which were attempts to explain the pattern of differences between states in dying from a particular cancer using regression analysis. Each connection is not only linear (straight line) in nature but is also "independent" after accounting for the effect of the others items in the model.

CONNECTED ITEMS

1. Earth Magnetism

As we drive north in the US, death rates from these cancers go up. This first group is best explained by the increasing strength of the Earth's magnetic field (as we drive north). (That small increases in the size of the magnetic field might harm human health is a new possibility raised by this research).

> All cancer deaths except lung (more deaths)
> Non-Hodgkins lymphoma (more deaths)
> Adult leukemia (more deaths)
> Prostate cancer (more deaths)

2. Ultraviolet

As we drive north in the US, death rates from this second group of cancers go up as well. This group is most closely linked to the gradual weakening in the intensity of the sun's ultraviolet that reaches the ground. (That insufficiently strong ultraviolet might play a role in dying from certain cancers is, generally speaking, a reversal of accepted notions).

> Lung cancer (weaker sun, more deaths)
> Melanoma skin cancer (weaker sun, more deaths)
> Urinary tract cancer (including bladder) (more deaths)
> Ovarian cancer (more deaths)
> Uterine cancer (more deaths)

3. Dentist

Not visiting the dentist often enough (perhaps an indicator of not being diligent enough in cleaning one's teeth at home) is linked with higher death rates from these cancers.

> Colon cancer (more deaths)
> Cervical cancer (more deaths)

VISITING the dentist is linked with this cancer (strangely)

> Uterine cancer (more deaths)

4. Dog

Living with a dog appears linked with more deaths from certain cancers. The more households in a state with a dog, the higher the death rate from the cancers listed below. (It makes me sad to include this unsettling finding).

> All cancer deaths except lung (more deaths)
> Melanoma skin cancer (more deaths)
> Adult leukemia (more deaths)

5. Smoking

Smoking tobacco cigarettes is linked with a higher death rate from two specific cancers as well as all cancer deaths.

> Colon cancer (more deaths)
> All cancer deaths (more deaths)
> [Lung cancer in alternative model not shown (more deaths)]

6. Air Pollution

Particle air pollution, also called particulate matter 2.5 microns, is tiny pieces of dirt (carbon) in the air so small that we cannot see them. More such dirt in the air in the downtown of the state's largest city over the course of the year is linked with a higher death rate from these cancers.

> Breast cancer (more deaths)
> Uterine cancer (more deaths)

7. Rain

The more inches of rain over the year in the largest city of the state, the higher the death rate from these cancers.

    All cancer deaths (more deaths)
    All cancer deaths except lung (more deaths)

8. Wine

The more wine consumed over the year, the higher the death rate from this cancer. (For this connection, all wine of various colors is grouped together).

    Pancreatic cancer among women (more deaths)

9. Height

The shorter the average height (of women) in a state, the higher the death rate from this cancer.

    Stomach cancer (more deaths)

The shorter the average height (of men) in a state, the higher the death rate from this cancer.

    Liver cancer among men (more deaths)

10. Frequent Sex

Having sex four times a week (perhaps suggesting multiple partners?) is linked with this cancer.

    Liver cancer among men (more deaths)

11. Elevation

Living at lower elevation (such as sea level). As you drive down from the mountains to the ocean, death rates from this cancer increase.

    Pancreatic cancer among women (more deaths)

DEMOGRAPHIC (PEOPLE) CHARACTERISTICS RELATED TO CANCER

12. College

The more people in the state who have attended college (even without getting a degree), the less likely people are to die from this cancer.

    Lung cancer (FEWER deaths)

13. Blacks

The more African Americans in a state, the death rate from these cancers is higher. This probably means Blacks are more likely to die from them. (About 13 percent of the American population identifies as Black).

    Prostate cancer (more deaths)
    Cervical cancer (more deaths)
    Stomach cancer (more deaths)
    Liver cancer among men (more deaths)

14. Jews

The more Jews in a state, the death rate from cancer (of all types) is LOWER. This probably means that Jews are less likely to die from cancer. (About 2 percent of the American population is estimated to be Jewish).

    All cancer deaths (FEWER deaths)

15. Seniors

The more seniors in the state (age 65 plus), the more deaths from these cancers. There are three groupings here about older age. In this first one, "age" is the largest connection.

>   All cancer deaths (more deaths)
>   All cancer deaths except lung (more deaths)
>   Color cancer (more deaths)
>   Urinary tract cancer (mainly bladder) (more deaths)
>   Non-Hodgkins lymphoma (more deaths)
>   Adult leukemia (more deaths)
>   Prostate cancer (more deaths)
>   Ovarian cancer (more deaths)
>   Uterine cancer (more deaths)

In this second age grouping, it is also true that the more seniors in the state (age 65 plus), the more deaths from these cancers. "Age", here, however, is NOT the largest connection.

>   Breast cancer (more deaths)
>   Melanoma skin cancer (more deaths)
>   Cervical cancer (more deaths)

More seniors in the state (age 65 plus) is NOT linked as an item with the cancers in this third group.

>   Pancreatic cancer in women
>   Stomach cancer
>   (For Lung cancer, age does not appear in the model presented but the connection is probably there indirectly through college because older people are less likely to have attended).

Air pollution is connected with two cancers, breast and uterine, showing that its negative effect on human health extends beyond the lungs and beyond heart disease to now include cancer.

To the surprise of all, perhaps, rain is linked with cancer. While unclear why or how, I speculate that higher gamma radiation in the air might be the real culprit.

To my chagrin, drinking wine is connected with one deadly cancer: pancreatic.

Shorter height is linked with two cancers: stomach and liver, for reasons that are unclear.

Frequent sex, four times a week, is linked with one cancer, perhaps evidence that liver cancer is first and foremost the long term result of the acquisition of a sexually transmitted virus.

Lastly, elevation appears to be a factor with one cancer: pancreatic, with living "low", near sea level, being linked with dying from this cancer.

For the four "people" items, percent Black is a noticeable part of the cancer story with several cancers. It is probably the case that Blacks are more likely to die of certain cancers when compared with the population as a whole. These include cervical, stomach and liver cancer.

Percent Jewish is also part of the story with Jews probably less likely to die from cancer in general compared to the American population as a whole. This is probably due, in part, to the possibility that Jews are less likely to live in households with a dog.

Lastly is seniors, the size of the population that is age 65 and older, a major part of the cancer story. This is no surprise as, to a large degree, confirmed here, cancer is "a disease of aging". It was essential to include the well known connection as a prerequisite for looking further.

The role of older age is divided in Table 17-3 into three categories. The first is where older age is the main connection. The second is where age is present but is not the strongest connection. The third category is where older age does not appear as connected to those cancers in a large enough way to be discernible using this statistical method.

Exactly nineteen years ago, I realized that my mother, who had sinus cancer, was going to die after the cancer kept coming back. I set out to try and prevent that from happening. She surely deserved that I should try because she was a great mother whom I loved. Two years after, she did die.

Now all these years later, this is what I learned. While I didn't succeed in saving my mother's life, I kept on working thanks to the intrinsic motivation generated by my interest in the science questions themselves. Working on a dissertation over a long period of time taught me that I was able to continue working largely without outside reinforcement or rewards. Without this freedom, I can't imagine that the work would have been able to proceed, at least in the way that it did.

Hopefully, this information will move us forward a little bit with what we know about cancer. Maybe one day, some piece of information here will lead us to figure something out which might help to save other good people. (August 10, 2016, 4:11 PM).

Chapter 18. The Eight "Northern" Cancers - a Meta Analysis. Is it Ultraviolet or Geomagnetism?

The concluding chapter was written. I thought I was done. Then I realized for about the first time the import of a recurring pattern for many of the cancers - north. There are actually eight kinds of cancer with this death pattern. As we drive north, more people die.

On the east coast of the United States, Interstate 95 runs from Florida up to Maine. We can imagine a hypothetical drive from Key West Florida to Bar Harbor Maine. After accounting for other factors, the same geographic pattern asserts itself for all eight of these cancers. The more north we drive, the more people die from these cancers. The same is true on the West Coast and in the middle of the country.

These eight northern cancers include lung, melanoma, ovarian, uterine, urinary, lymphoma, adult leukemia and prostate. Why is this? I give two answers to this question based on the model results for each cancer.

Five of these eight "northern" cancers are linked with insufficiently strong ultraviolet in sunlight reaching the ground at "solar noon", when the sun is highest in the sky of the day. As the sun gets weaker on the way north, more people die from this group of five cancers: lung, melanoma, ovarian, uterine and cancer of the urinary tract (including bladder).

For another three of these "northern" cancers, the individual model results point to another environmental item that changes on the drive north. Earth magnetism keeps getting stronger along the way. These three "northern" cancers are linked to higher geomagnetism - lymphoma, adult leukemia and prostate.

An unpleasant thought has been in the background for a long while. The regression method allows us to test competing possible explanations for this northern pattern including ultraviolet and geomagnetism. This is very standard.

In this case, however, both competitors - ultraviolet and geomagnetism - are highly correlated with each other at the level of about .9 (the highest being 1). In such a situation, both possibilities, quite obviously, could not be in the same model because a high intercorrelation violates the rules of the method. This could lead to misleading results. The regression method helped us to decide which of the two worked better. This was reported in the original model for each individual cancer in previous chapters and summarized in the two categories above.

The unpleasant thought is as follows. As I mention in the introduction, the model results are an imperfect representation of "reality" for various reasons. One example is that results can change based on other items in the model. A second broad obvious category is "error" in the process of converting an idea into number form for testing.

Might it not be possible that "in reality", there is one environmental factor rather than two that explains the northern pattern of all of these cancers? If this were the case, which would it be, of the two we have identified?

It is difficult to view reality directly in the context of this project. We can only view it indirectly and imperfectly from the results of the statistical models and their analysis.

Nevertheless, in this chapter, I endeavor to clarify the matter as much as possible by doing three new sets of analyses.

In the first, I add the ultraviolet cancers together and then do a new model for them. In the second, I do the same for the geomagnetism-linked cancers. In the third, I combine all the northern cancers together and do a new model for these. Then, I attempt to reach a conclusion about all eight northern cancers regarding which environmental factor might best account for the pattern.

Of course, this is not the first time here that death rates from different cancers have been combined together. In the first chapter, we discussed all kinds of cancer together while, in the chapter that followed it, we took a look at all cancers with the exception of the largest one, lung cancer.

What is different in this case is that, here, we use the death rate lists from the best models for each disease. They are not all from the same year. Thus, adding them together is a rather "Frankenstein" creation. I justify this decision in the following way.

First, it makes a certain sense, because the constructs are linked thematically with a "northern" pattern (which becomes apparent only after controls). Second, they are linked to sub-themes of a connection with either the diminished intensity of ultraviolet in sunlight or increased geomagnetism. Third, the individual death lists used for each cancer happened to yield the most successful model. This suggests relatively little error in those particular lists. Fourth, it is my impression that the death rate pattern between states for these cancers does not change very much from one year to the next over the course of years not too far from each other.

In Table 18-1, I add the death rate numbers for each cancer together that are linked with insufficient ultraviolet. These five cancers are lung in Table 3-1, melanoma in Table 6-1, ovarian in Table 12-1, uterine in Table 13-1 and urinary (majority bladder) in Table 7-1. The statistical software program does this easily for each state. I will give the example of New York, the state of my birth, looking up the value from each death rate list.

For New York, the death rate from lung cancer is 59.6 deaths per hundred thousand. For melanoma in the best model, it is 3.1 deaths per hundred thousand. For ovarian cancer, it is 8.5 deaths. For uterine cancer, it is 4.9 deaths, and for urinary tract cancer (including bladder), it is 8.7 deaths.

These add to 84.8 deaths and that is the number for New York on the new combined item for the "not strong enough uv" cancers in Table 18-1 called [can5uv]. This obviously stands for the five cancers linked to not strong enough ultraviolet.

Next are the remaining "northern" cancers where there are more deaths on the trip north which are most strongly linked to the OTHER environmental factor which changes as we head north - the strength of the Earth's magnetic field. This gets stronger along the way (north). These three remaining northern cancers include Non-Hodgkin's lymphoma, adult leukemia and prostate. Again here, we add the lists together telling the program to add the following three lists of numbers for each state.

The death rate list for lymphoma is from Table 8-1. Adult Leukemia is from Table 10-1 and prostate is from Table 11-1. Taking the value for New York as an example of one state, for lymphoma, the death rate is 6.9 deaths per hundred thousand people. For adult leukemia, it is 9.2 deaths and for prostate, it is 11.5 deaths. This adds to 27.6 death, the value for New York for this new grouping of deaths from cancers linked with Earth magnetism that is too strong. I named it [can3geo] which stands for the three northern cancers that are linked with stronger geomagnetism as we drive north. This new list is found in Table 18-2.

Table 18-1.can5uv.

The five northern cancers added together that are linked to insufficiently strong ultraviolet: lung, urinary (bladder), melanoma, ovarian and uterine. Death rate per hundred thousand people.

State	Rate	State	Rate
Utah	39.2	Oregon	94.6
Colorado	60.0	Wisconsin	95.1
California	64.0	New Hampshire	95.8
Alaska	66.0	South Dakota	96.1
Hawaii	66.5	North Carolina	97.7
New Mexico	68.1	Louisiana	100.5
Texas	69.3	Vermont	100.5
District	72.0	South Carolina	100.8
Wyoming	73.2	Michigan	101.7
Idaho	75.6	Iowa	104.5
Arizona	78.0	Florida	105.0
Minnesota	80.6	Rhode Island	105.2
Georgia	80.7	Indiana	106.6
Washington	82.4	Pennsylvania	107.3
Maryland	83.4	Delaware	107.5
Nevada	83.5	Mississippi	107.8
New York	84.8	Alabama	108.4
Virginia	85.4	Oklahoma	110.8
New Jersey	85.7	Ohio	110.9
Connecticut	86.0	Missouri	111.6
North Dakota	89.9	Tennessee	112.5
Nebraska	91.1	Arkansas	119.0
Illinois	91.4	Maine	120.8
Massachusetts	92.2	Kentucky	128.3
Montana	93.3	West Virginia	130.3
Kansas	93.9		

Table 18-2. can3geo.

The three "northern" cancers that are linked with higher geomagnetism added together: lymphoma, adult leukemia and prostate. Death rates per hundred thousand people.

Alaska	16.1	Massachusetts	29.7
Texas	22.3	Connecticut	30.0
Utah	22.4	Vermont	30.0
Hawaii	22.7	Tennessee	30.0
Georgia	23.2	Michigan	30.1
Colorado	23.4	Kansas	30.3
Nevada	24.4	Indiana	30.6
California	24.6	Minnesota	30.9
Virginia	25.3	Rhode Island	30.9
New Mexico	25.9	Oklahoma	30.9
Maryland	26.0	Ohio	31.3
Mississippi	26.9	North Dakota	31.7
Washington	27.6	Nebraska	31.9
New York	27.6	Arkansas	31.9
Arizona	27.8	Alabama	32.0
North Car	27.8	Oregon	32.1
New Hampshire	28.1	Montana	32.5
New Jersey	28.3	Maine	32.8
Louisiana	28.4	Missouri	32.9
District	28.7	Florida	33.3
Illinois	28.7	Wisconsin	33.4
South Carolina	29.0	Iowa	33.9
Kentucky	29.1	West Virginia	33.9
Idaho	29.2	South Dakota	34.2
Delaware	29.2	Pennsylvania	34.4
Wyoming	29.4		

Lastly is the combination of all eight "northern" cancers which share in common the fact that this entire group has more deaths as we drive north in the United States. These cancers include the five linked with not strong enough ultraviolet: lung, melanoma, ovarian, uterine and urinary tract, as well as the three high geomagnetism ones: lymphoma, adult leukemia, and prostate.

Of course, we do not have to add each of the seven together because it is the same now to add the two larger groupings together, the numbers in Table 18-1 and Table 18-2. This last new meta item of all the northern cancers can be found in Table 18-3 called [can8nor3] which obviously stands for the combination of all eight northern cancers. (The number three at the end is the result of minor errors in the first two versions of the item). [It made sense to me to construct all of these new groupings now even though the analysis of Table 18-3 (with all eight cancers together) is presented much later in the chapter].

Using the state of New York again as an example, the death rate for the five insufficiently strong UV ones in Table 18-1 is 84.8. In Table 18-2, the New York death rate for the additional three geomagnetism-linked cancer is 27.6. This adds to a combined death rate for New York from all eight "northern" cancers of 112.4 deaths per hundred thousand. That is indeed the number for New York in Table 18-3 [can8nor3].

With these new combo items now in place, we are ready to do new models in order to see first if the earlier results from the individual models might be reconfirmed in the aggregate. Might there be a specific item that stands out from among the different ones in the original model? Then we can move to answer the grand question. Which "northern" environmental factor is stronger, (insufficiently intense) ultraviolet, or (higher) geomagnetism on the ground (in the largest city of the state).

The first meta model appears in Table 18-4 can5uv model. The result strongly confirms in a general way the conclusions from the separate models.

We can look more closely now at the results in Table 18-4, the meta model of the northern cancers linked with not strong enough ultraviolet. As usual, we look to the bottom box to check the correlation between the two items in the model. It is a very low number [-.08, not significant (no stars)], this being a good thing. Glancing at the bottom line, there is a very large correlation between attending college and (not) dying from these five cancers (-.830**). Of course, this connection is in a negative direction. More people in a state who have attended college, fewer deaths from these five northern cancers.

Table 18-3. can8nor3.

The eight "northern" cancers added together: the five linked to insufficiently strong ultraviolet: lung, urinary (bladder), melanoma, ovarian, and uterine, as well as the additional three linked with higher geomagnetism: lymphoma, adult leukemia and prostate. Death rates per hundred thousand people.

Utah	61.6		North Carolina	125.5
Alaska	82.1		Montana	125.8
Colorado	83.4		Oregon	126.7
California	88.6		Wisconsin	128.5
Hawaii	89.2		Louisiana	128.9
Texas	91.6		South Carolina	129.8
New Mexico	94.0		South Dakota	130.3
District	100.7		Vermont	130.5
Wyoming	102.6		Michigan	131.8
Georgia	103.9		Mississippi	134.7
Idaho	104.8		Rhode Island	136.1
Arizona	105.8		Delaware	136.7
Nevada	107.9		Indiana	137.2
Maryland	109.4		Florida	138.3
Washington	110.0		Iowa	138.4
Virginia	110.7		Alabama	140.4
Minnesota	111.5		Oklahoma	141.7
New York	112.4		Pennsylvania	141.7
New Jersey	114.0		Ohio	142.2
Connecticut	116.0		Tennessee	142.5
Illinois	120.1		Missouri	144.5
North Dakota	121.6		Arkansas	150.9
Massachusetts	121.9		Maine	153.6
Nebraska	123.0		Kentucky	157.4
New Hampshire	123.9		West Virginia	164.2
Kansas	124.2			

More interesting perhaps is the possible link between ultraviolet [UVI0614] (UV Index in the largest city between the years 2006 and 2014) and dying from these five cancers. There is no significant connection (-.201, not significant). Apparently, we must first control for the huge effect of college before this connection between insufficiently intense ultraviolet and dying from these cancers can come into view.

Moving up now to the top box, we see that the entire model has an Adjusted R Square of .751. The model as a whole, consisting of attending college and how strong the ultraviolet is that reaches the ground around noon time in the largest city of the state, explains just a tad more than 75 percent of the pattern or three quarters.

The final model itself appears in the middle box. Starting with the significance, which is an indication of how solid the connections are, the result is quite solid. While the Sig. value is .000, not unusual in this research, what stands out in the t column is the value for the link between college and not dying from these five northern cancers, a 12, way above the needed 2. For ultraviolet [uvi0614], the t value is -3.79, suggesting that the link between ultraviolet and not dying from these five northern cancers is also sufficiently solid.

Apparently, the aggregation together might have strengthened further the impact of college on this group of cancers. To repeat the observations from the chapter on lung cancer, the powerful result linking attendance at college with fewer deaths is partly the result of the fact that more older people in a state over age 65 is linked with fewer people who have attended college. This is probably because going to college was less common years ago when this age group was young. As we all know, dying is linked with older age and this is particularly true for cancer (as a generalization). Of course, older age could not be in this same model because it is too closely connected with (not attending) college thus breaking the technical rules of the method.

The other possible explanation of the huge impact of college is smoking, also too closely linked with college to be in the model. There is a negative connection between the two, with the percent of people who smoke every day in the state going down the higher the percent of people who have attended college.

It is possible to build a variety of models for these five cancers. In the end, I chose this model in Table 18-4 partly because the connection between the items is so low, a technical advantage implying that the result is clean. Whether or not this model illuminates "reality" better than other possibilities is unclear to me.

The Beta column gives us information about the relative strength of each item compared to the others.

Table 18-4 The Model for the five northern cancers added together that are linked to insufficiently strong ultraviolet in sunlight: lung, urinary (bladder), melanoma, ovarian and uterine.

Model Summary

Model	R	R Square	Adjusted R Square	Std. Error of the Estimate
1	.872[a]	.761	.751	9.1703

a. Predictors: (Constant), UVI0614, SUMCOLIG

Coefficients[a]

Model		Unstandardized Coefficients		Standardized Coefficients	t	Sig.
		B	Std. Error	Beta		
1	(Constant)	216.410	10.363		20.882	.000
	SUMCOLIG	-2.354	.196	-.851	-12.014	.000
	UVI0614	-3.315	.875	-.269	-3.790	.000

a. Dependent Variable: CAN5UV

Correlations

		SUMCOLIG	UVI0614	CAN5UV
SUMCOLIG	Pearson Correlation	1	-.080	-.830**
	Sig. (2-tailed)	.	.578	.000
	N	51	51	51
UVI0614	Pearson Correlation	-.080	1	-.201
	Sig. (2-tailed)	.578	.	.158
	N	51	51	51
CAN5UV	Pearson Correlation	-.830**	-.201	1
	Sig. (2-tailed)	.000	.158	.
	N	51	51	51

**. Correlation is significant at the 0.01 level (2-tailed).

We can add the two values together without the decimals and signs (851+269=1120). Of the portion of the pattern that the model explains (about three quarters), college explains (851/1120=.76) about 76 percent. Ultraviolet clarifies (269/1120=.24) about 24 percent of this explained portion of the pattern.

We can now slightly adjust these numbers to view them in terms of their part of the ENTIRE explanation, the part of the total pattern that the model succeeds to explain (three quarters) and the remaining quarter it fails to explain. Using the Adjusted R Square, we know that 1120/.751=x/1. 1120=.751x. X=1120/.751. X=1491.34, the new denominator for the total explanation. For college, this is 851/1491.34=.57. Of the total explanation, attending college explains about 57 percent.

For ultraviolet, it is 269/1491.34=.18. Of the total pattern for these UV-diminished cancers with this northern pattern of more deaths, ultraviolet explains about 18 percent of the total explanation. At this point, I will refrain from constructing a "best view" of this combined group of cancers saving this exercise for the final aggregate version.

I have two concluding comments about this cancer group linked with ultraviolet. First is the technical detail that the ultraviolet measure that worked best for this meta model was the updated one [uv0614]. This includes yearly ultraviolet reaching the ground in the largest city of the state over the course of nine year, from 2006-2014. I was very pleased that this new measure, constructed by NOAA's Craig Long relatively recently, was able to play a role in confirming the validity of the earlier work. There, a link between certain cancers and insufficiently intense ultraviolet (based on the pattern of death rates between the states) was suggested. As I have stated earlier as well, the results here are my own and do not reflect any endorsement by either Mr. Long or NOAA.

Second, the success here in being able to construct this model from this new aggregate set of numbers provides additional evidence to support the possibility that ultraviolet might be the better explanation compared with geomagnetism for this particular group of five northern cancers. Once again, this group includes lung, melanoma, ovarian, urinary (bladder) and uterine. The two possibilities were tested against each other using this final model and ultraviolet came out as significantly related to deaths from these five cancer. Geomagnetism was not significantly related when both were tested in this same model.

Now, we are ready to move to the geomagnetism-linked northern cancers, which include Non-Hodgkin's lymphoma, adult leukemia and prostate. In the original models, all three are linked with Earth magnetism. Here, when the three cancers in this group are aggregated (added) together, would the model confirm a link with geomagnetism? Might it be possible to show a link with ultraviolet as well? If so, this could lead to the tantalizing conclusion that perhaps ultraviolet was the "genuine" environmental factor responsible for the northern pattern even for these cancers.

In this aggregated form, it turned out to be easy to create a model that confirms the link between these cancers and Earth magnetism. As in the original models, the higher the Earth magnetism measured on the ground (as we travel north), the more deaths from this group of cancers. While I decided not to show this model, not to select it as the most interesting one, it consists of two items: a higher percent of the population of the state in the older age category of age 65 (more deaths) and higher Earth magnetism [geomag08], (more deaths). While the result is overall, clear and powerful, it does suffer from one minor blemish, a small correlation between the items (-.144, not significant).

At the eleventh hour, I decided to double check the main theme here, using the above model to test the alternative possibility that these cancers might actually be related instead to the diminished intensity of ultraviolet as we drive north. To my surprise, it was also very easy to build such an alternative model which is the one I decided to present as the most intriguing result.

This model for [can3geo] with ultraviolet is presented in Table 18-5. The model has two items: older age [age65in6] and ultraviolet [uvi0614]. The higher the percent of the state population in this older age category, the more deaths from this group of cancers. The lower the intensity of ultraviolet in sunlight reaching the ground around noon in the largest city of the state, the more deaths there are from this group of cancers.

Looking now at Table 18-5, we start with the bottom box as usual to see a very low intercorrelation between the items (.090, not significant). This score being lower than the geomagnetism model (-.144) is one reason I thought this to be a slightly better model. The bottom line shows a huge link between older age and dying from this group of cancers (+.848**). There is little connection between the death rate from these cancers and ultraviolet (-.243).

Table 18-5 The model for the three northern cancers added together thatwere previously linked with higher geomagnetism (lymphoma, adult leukemia and prostate): a possible role for insufficiently strong ultraviolet.

Model Summary

Model	R	R Square	Adjusted R Square	Std. Error of the Estimate
1	.907[a]	.822	.815	1.6084

a. Predictors: (Constant), UVI0614, AGE65IN6

Coefficients[a]

Model		Unstandardized Coefficients		Standardized Coefficients	t	Sig.
		B	Std. Error	Beta		
1	(Constant)	8.346	1.848		4.517	.000
	AGE65IN6	1.958	.137	.877	14.339	.000
	UVI0614	-.809	.154	-.322	-5.267	.000

a. Dependent Variable: CAN3GEO

Correlations

		AGE65IN6	UVI0614	CAN3GEO
AGE65IN6	Pearson Correlation	1	.090	.848**
	Sig. (2-tailed)	.	.531	.000
	N	51	51	51
UVI0614	Pearson Correlation	.090	1	-.243
	Sig. (2-tailed)	.531	.	.085
	N	51	51	51
CAN3GEO	Pearson Correlation	.848**	-.243	1
	Sig. (2-tailed)	.000	.085	.
	N	51	51	51

**. Correlation is significant at the 0.01 level (2-tailed).

Apparently, the large effect of older age must first be accounted for in the final model before this connection reveals itself. The top box shows the Adjusted R Square of the model as a whole is .815, meaning that the model explains 81.5 percent of the death pattern between all the states.

Lastly is the final model itself found in the middle box of Table 18-5. The two right boxes show strong, solid results with the Sig. t of both items .000. The t value is also large for both, having to be over 2. For age, it is a very large 14 plus and for ultraviolet, it is over 5.

The Beta column shows the relative size of each item. The effect of age is much larger. First we find the size of each item as a portion of the explanation that the model uncovered. We add both values together in the Beta column (without signs or decimals): 877+322=1199, now our denominator. The portion of older age is 877/1199=.73 or 73 percent of the explanation uncovered in the model. For ultraviolet, it is 322/1199=.269 or about 27 percent of the explanation.

It is perhaps more interesting to know how much of the total possible explanation for death rates from these cancers might be explained by each item. We know that the model explains 81.5 percent of that total. For this, we create a new denominator using the Adjusted R Square. 1199/.815=x/1. 1199=.815x. 1199/.815=x. x=1471.2.

For the size of the age effect as a portion of the total possible explanation, it is 877/1471.2=.596 or 59.6 percent, close to 57 percent. For ultraviolet, it is 322/1471.2=.219 or about 22 percent of the total explanation, a little more than a fifth. Like with the last grouping, we will skip the further representation of the result in a predicted death rate list saving this exercise for the final amalgamation that follows.

What can we conclude from this aggregate look at the three northern cancers that were, earlier, linked with Earth magnetism? At this higher level of aggregation, we see two things. One is a confirmation that Earth magnetism still could be a "genuine" environmental factor that is responsible for the northern pattern of these three cancers (including lymphoma, adult leukemia and prostate). This is the clear result of an earlier model described but not shown above. Yet, in the end, I decided to present another alternative model, quite successful as well, showing a connection between insufficiently strong ultraviolet and deaths from this group of cancers.

In the context of the question posed here, this result in Table 18-5 is most intriguing. It raises the possibility that these three additional cancers might actually have their northern pattern (more deaths as we travel north in the United States) as the result of a connection with the weaker sun the further north we go. Due to the success of both models and hence, both possibilities, we cannot know for sure, at this time, which might be closer to "truth". Nevertheless, this aggregation moves the matter forward considerably by raising the possibility that even these cancers might actually be "northern" because of a connection to the weaker sun.

The last test is what could be called the meta-meta model combining both groupings of these northern cancers together. These include the five cancers linked with insufficiently strong ultraviolet even in their original separate models. These are lung, melanoma, ovarian, uterine and urinary tract (including bladder). These are now added together with the additional three cancers that were linked with too high Earth magnetism in the original models. These include lymphoma, adult leukemia and prostate. (To repeat, adding together the two previous meta groups in Tables 18-1 and 18-2 is the same as adding each of the eight cancers together from scratch).

This final meta construct of the eight northern cancers together can be seen in Table 18-3 (placed several pages back where it is first mentioned). It is called [can8nor3], for the eight northern cancers (together) - sharing a similar pattern of more deaths as we travel north. (The final "3" is merely a record that this is the third try to get the item correct). This northern pattern is not apparent from the list in Table 18-3 but becomes apparent in time after controls are introduced for the other single item (in this case) which, itself, has a big effect on the pattern in these numbers.

From looking at Table 18-3, Utah is the state with the lowest starting death rate for these eight northern cancers with a rate of about 62 deaths. West Virginia is the last state on the list with the highest death rate of about 164 deaths. The "variation" is quite substantial. If the rate in Utah is set at 1, the rate in West Virginia is larger by how much? $61.6/1=164.2x$. $61.6x=164.2$. $x=164.2/61.6=2.67$. The death rate from these eight cancers in the highest state is 2.67 times larger than the lowest death rate state, between two and three times larger.

What will prove to be the decisive factor which best explains these cancers when united together in this higher level of aggregation? Will it be the insufficiently intense ultraviolet in sunlight as we travel north, or the increased strength of the planet's magnetic field?

The answer can be found in Table 18-6, the [can8nor] model, which we will now review patiently as has been the pattern throughout. First is the quick preview summary. The model has two items, attending college (fewer deaths from these eight northern cancers) and ultraviolet (also fewer deaths the stronger it is). The list for attending college by state can be found back in Chapter 3 about lung cancer, Table 3-2. The list for the average intensity of ultraviolet reaching the ground in the largest city of each state (using the UV Index from NOAA) can be found on Table 3-3.

Looking now at Table 18-6, we start with the bottom box to make sure the correlation between the two items is not too high, a technical problem which can lead to erroneous results. We see that the link between college [sumcolig] and ultraviolet [uvi0614] is, thankfully, very low at -.080. This is one of the reasons I chose the model. The last row shows a link between college and these cancers of -.811**, a large starting connection between going to college and fewer deaths from these cancers. The link between these cancers and ultraviolet [uvi0614] is low and not significant. This main result, apparently, only appears in the final model after accounting for the huge effect of college. The top box shows an Adjusted R square of .726 meaning that the model as a whole accounts for 72.6 percent of the total pattern in death rates between states from this grouping of eight northern cancers.

Now we move to the middle box which contains the main model. Starting on the right with the two boxes which provide information about the statistical significance of these connections, The Sig. value for both is .000, very good. The t value for college is very large in size, over 11. For ultraviolet [uvi0614], it is around 3.8, solidly above the needed 2.

The Beta column shows the relative size of each effect and its contribution to the total part of the explanation that is captured by the model. A cursory look reveals that the effect of college is much larger. To figure the size of each item, we add both Betas together (ignoring signs and decimals): 822+284=1117, which we use as our denominator. College accounts for 822/1117=.736 or 73.6 percent of the explanation that the model uncovered. Ultraviolet accounts for 284/1117=.254 or 25.4 percent of that explanation.

Table 18-6 Model for the eight northern cancers added all together: the possible role of insufficiently strong ultraviolet in sunlight. The eight northern cancers include lung, urinary(bladder), melanoma, ovarian, uterine, Non-Hodgkins lymphoma, adult leukemia and prostate.

Model Summary

Model	R	R Square	Adjusted R Square	Std. Error of the Estimate
1	.859[a]	.737	.726	11.0626

a. Predictors: (Constant), UVI0614, SUMCOLIG

Coefficients[a]

Model		Unstandardized Coefficients		Standardized Coefficients	t	Sig.
		B	Std. Error	Beta		
1	(Constant)	262.741	12.502		21.016	.000
	SUMCOLIG	-2.655	.236	-.833	-11.232	.000
	UVI0614	-4.033	1.055	-.284	-3.822	.000

a. Dependent Variable: CAN8NOR3

Correlations

		SUMCOLIG	UVI0614	CAN8NOR3
SUMCOLIG	Pearson Correlation	1	-.080	-.811**
	Sig. (2-tailed)	.	.578	.000
	N	51	51	51
UVI0614	Pearson Correlation	-.080	1	-.217
	Sig. (2-tailed)	.578	.	.126
	N	51	51	51
CAN8NOR3	Pearson Correlation	-.811**	-.217	1
	Sig. (2-tailed)	.000	.126	.
	N	51	51	51

**. Correlation is significant at the 0.01 level (2-tailed).

More interesting is to know the size as part of the total explanation knowing that the model accounts for about 73 percent of that total. We use the Adjusted R Square (.726) to calculate the new denominator: .726/1117=1/x. .726x=1117. X=1117/.726=1538.6. For college, the size of its effect as a portion of the total possible explanation is (833/1538.6=.541 or) 54.1 percent, over half. For ultraviolet, it is (284/1538.6=.185 or) 18.5 percent of the total possible explanation, a little under a fifth.

Another way to confirm the size of the main ultraviolet finding is by creating a "best view" version of death rates from all eight cancers after accounting for the huge impact of going to college. Of course, the result in this new predicted death rate list will have the same ordering as ultraviolet [uvi0614] (but in reverse because the stronger the ultraviolet, the lower the death rate from these eight cancers). This is because, using the model in Table 18-6, we are only allowing one item to vary, ultraviolet [uvi0614].

The impact of college is accounted for and held to the side by using its mean (average) value for all of the states together. We do this by using the equation in the middle box of Table 18-6 and letting the statistical program "solve" it for each state, this time holding constant the effect of college. What results is a transformed version of the original death rate list in Table 18-3, which, itself, is a combined version of all eight original death rate lists for these cancers.

Referring now to the equation in Table 18-6 (in the B column), it is 262.741 – [2.655 * (times) the mean value for college, 45.422 (percent)] – [4.033 * (times) uvi0614, the value for each state for ultraviolet over the nine year period]. I will run this now.

I call this the "best view" of death rates from these eight cancers can8norl, which stands for cancer 8 north list. It can be found in Table 18-7. Compared with the original death rate combined list of the eight cancers in Table 18-3, Table 18-7 represents a more interesting view of the pattern.

While the connection with going to college is nice to know, we are more focused here on the role of the environment and it is only after setting aside the matter of college, done in Table 18-7, that we can begin to see the impact of not strong enough ultraviolet in sunlight as we travel north.

Table 18-7 can8norl. Cancer 8 north list.

Predicted deaths from the eight northern cancers per hundred thousand people after holding constant the large effect of college but allowing ultraviolet to vary (represented by the UV index in the largest city of the state over a nine year period). The eight cancers added together include death rates from lung, melanoma, ovarian, uterine, urinary (including bladder), Non-Hodgkins lymphoma, adult leukemia and prostate.

Hawaii	97.4	New Jersey	123.6
Florida	107.9	Delaware	123.6
Louisiana	113.1	West Virginia	123.6
California	113.9	Nebraska	124.0
New Mexico	113.9	Indiana	124.0
Alabama	113.9	New York	124.4
Texas	114.3	Montana	124.4
Arizona	114.3	Pennsylvania	124.4
Mississippi	116.3	Iowa	124.8
Nevada	116.7	Connecticut	125.2
South Carolina	116.7	Illinois	125.2
Georgia	117.9	Massachusetts	125.2
Colorado	118.8	South Dakota	125.2
Utah	119.2	Rhode Island	125.2
Oklahoma	119.6	Ohio	125.2
Arkansas	119.6	Wisconsin	125.6
Wyoming	120.0	New Hampshire	126.0
Tennessee	120.0	Michigan	126.0
Virginia	120.4	Minnesota	126.4
North Carolina	120.4	North Dakota	126.4
Kansas	121.2	Maine	126.4
Idaho	122.4	Oregon	127.6
Missouri	122.8	Vermont	127.6
Kentucky	122.8	Washington	128.0
District	123.6	Alaska	134.5
Maryland	123.6		

The lowest predicted death rate from the eight northern cancers is in Hawaii with some 97 deaths. The highest is in the most northern state, Alaska, with about 135 deaths. Compared with the lowest predicted death rate, how much larger is the highest rate? 97.4/1=134.5/x/ 97.4x=134.5. x=134.5/97.4. x=1.38. The predicted death rate from these cancers is 38 percent larger in the state of Alaska compared with the state of Hawaii on account of the less intense ultraviolet that reaches the ground on an average day over the nine year period.

While the earlier conclusion was that ultraviolet accounted for 18 percent of the total pattern in death rates, this result suggests that the actual difference in death rates due to the difference in ultraviolet between the smallest and largest values is larger, some 38 percent. Perhaps it is due to the fact that both values are outliers (quite distant from typical death rate values on the list) thus exaggerating the impact.

Now we are ready for the analysis because we could have an exciting finding here. In the original models, quite belatedly, I detected a similar northern pattern for these eight cancers. After controls were introduced, there was the same geographic pattern for the country as a whole. As we drove north from Key West Florida to Bar Harbor Maine, more people (per population size) kept dying from these cancers. The result suggests that this pattern is generally true anywhere in the United States, including for the west coast, driving from San Diego California to Seattle Washington (which I have also done).

This combination of death rates from eight kinds of cancer in Table 18-3 has a mean (average) value of 121.435 deaths. For death rates from cancer (in general) in 2010-2012, the mean yearly death rate is 248.122. While not exact because the years do not match up, we can divide the mean death number for the eight cancers by the mean for the total death rate from all cancers to get an approximate idea of what portion these eight northern cancers are of all deaths from cancer. 121.435/248.122=.4894.

Death rates from these eight northern cancers represent about 48.9 percent of all cancer death rates. If these eight northern cancers represent almost half of all deaths from cancer in a given year, coming up with a possible explanation for this pattern might represent a step forward.

We are not quite finished, however, due to the confusion engendered by conflicting results. With five of the eight northern cancers, there is no such problem. For lung, melanoma, urinary (including bladder), ovarian, and uterine, the result is clear. The original individual models in the various chapters pointed to insufficiently strong ultraviolet as the best explanation. When these were added all together, this connection to ultraviolet was confirmed a second time to a satisfactory degree. In the final aggregation, when all eight northern cancers were added together, this connection with ultraviolet was confirmed a third time.

The situation is different for the three remaining cancers, Non-Hodgkin's lymphoma, adult leukemia and prostate. The original models in the earlier chapters pointed to a connection with Earth magnetism. When these three were added together and a new model was made, the result was inconclusive. While such a link with stronger Earth magnetism was easily confirmed (in a model not shown), an intriguing different possibility revealed itself for the first time.

In aggregated form, it became clear that perhaps this northern pattern was the result of a connection with weaker ultraviolet in sunlight as we drove north. This is the model I presented in Table 18-5 [can3geo]. Lastly, in the higher level of aggregation, when all eight northern cancers were added together, the result was more definitive. For all eight cancers together, ultraviolet was the clear "winner". It provided the best explanation overall.

Where does this leave us in terms of our assessment of the three cancers whose individual models pointed to Earth magnetism but when added together, aggregated models pointed eventually to ultraviolet? Each reader is free to assess these conflicting results in the manner which makes the most sense to them.

On the one hand, the individual model for each allows for a strong statement about the link between each of the three cancers and Earth magnetism. On the other hand, adding together the death rate lists used in the very strongest models for each cancer confers added power to the analysis. I presume that this is partly the result of the larger sizes of the death rates.

It should be clear that my own assessment is that the evidence as a whole points to the explanation of ultraviolet for this northern pattern for all eight of these cancers. I suspect that this added power of the aggregated models yields a result that is more "true". The sun gets weaker on the drive north together with its ultraviolet portion and it is this weakening that is linked in some manner with more deaths from these eight cancers.

I have generally tried to refrain from commenting about the specifics of cancer hoping that I have sufficiently identified such thoughts as speculation by a non-expert. Nevertheless, I wish that the reader would permit me to mention two ideas which seem to follow from the statistical analysis of these death rates.

First, if these eight cancers, after controls, exhibit the same geographic pattern of deaths – north – then I wonder if they are actually close to the same thing showing up in different parts of the body. Second, if such happens to be the case, I suspect that the same treatment might work for them all.

Chapter 19. Why Stop with Eight Cancers? Another Look at All Deaths from Cancer with the Exception of Lung Cancer. This Larger Group Might also Connect with Insufficiently Strong Ultraviolet in Sunlight.

Again, I figured I was done. Last night, however, I thought it now time to go back to all deaths from cancer with the exception of lung cancer from Chapter 2. At the beginning of this research, I started looking at all cancer deaths from the same source in the government chart. It was death rates from cancer of all types.

I am not sure whether this was an aggregation of the cancer death rates listed in the Health Data Interactive chart only or whether it also included those deaths from more esoteric (rare) cancers not included in their chart. I presume this list of all deaths from cancer is just that, the second option, including cancer of all kinds.

For Chapter 2, I separated out lung cancer on a hunch that this biggest of all cancers in terms of deaths (27.7 percent) might be distinctive. While my reasons for this decision are unclear, even to myself, at the very least, there is the special role of cigarette smoking in harming the lungs specifically, leading not only to lung cancer but also non-cancer lung disease called COPD, also a leading cause of death.

These numbers had the certain advantage compared to the ones I added together in the last chapter because they were surely all from the same set of years. Here, it was cancer death rates in 2010-2012 averaged into a yearly rate.

This solved the possible "Frankenstein" problem in the last chapter, combining original death rate lists which produced the most successful models even though they might be from different years. While I was fine with this decision, I was not sure how others might view it given its unusual nature.

After the excitement of the last chapter showing that the best explanation for the eight "northern" cancers when aggregated together turned out to be insufficiently strong ultraviolet, I was motivated to check further. These eight cancers accounted for some 49 percent of total deaths from cancer. Perhaps this finding about ultraviolet might even be larger?

I started quite from scratch to model death rates in 2010-2012 from cancer of all kinds with the exception of lung cancer, a list called [canolung] in Chapter 2, which is short for cancer no lung. As is typical, I was beset by many problems involving an improper link between the items I tested (multicollinearity). I also had a variety of choices regarding which model to present.

One disappointment was that geomagnetism worked better than ultraviolet with this set of numbers. This appears to conflict with my general conclusion that ultraviolet was the stronger explanation for the "northern" pattern of deaths from various groupings of cancer. For this reason, while I have, nevertheless, chosen to present an "ultraviolet" model, it cannot be used here independently to demonstrate that ultraviolet is the stronger explanation of the two.

Over a day and a half, I tried to figure out the best way to proceed, changing my mind back and forth while pondering the results of various models. The breakthrough toward my final decision came when I realized something about the original model in Chapter 2 for cancer without lung, deaths in 2010-2012. Even then, the finding that the pattern was linked with geomagnetism was an early confirmation of the northern pattern, more deaths from cancer without lung the more north we go. Of course, back at that time, I had not yet realized its import.

The model I chose as final is a reaffirmation of that northern pattern of dying from cancer (without lung). This simpler model will be presented only after my extensive commentary, a different format than previous chapters, given the possible implications of this result.

The upcoming model makes even clearer that this northern pattern extends now past the eight northern cancers in the last chapter to all cancers (except lung). This raises the total of cancer deaths from some 49 percent to 72.3 percent (minus the 27.7 percent of cancer deaths from lung cancer during those years).

Furthermore, even though lung is analyzed separately in Chapter 3, I reminded myself that, for lung cancer as well, this northern pattern is confirmed. More north, more deaths. Taken together, this northern pattern seems to hold for all cancers deaths when the death rates from individual kinds of cancer are aggregated together. Good Lord.

This research, then, provides evidence that death from "cancer" in general expresses the same geographic pattern of "north", more deaths as we travel north. This becomes apparent in the various models after setting aside other items with which different cancers are connected, one example being the large effect of older age.

The model for cancer no lung [canolung] will soon confirm the northern pattern in a different, simpler model (compared to the fuller one in Chapter 2). The question remains open regarding which idea of the two competing ones provides the best overall explanation for "north".

Which environmental factor best explains this pattern given that there are two leading candidates, both of which change as we travel north. Is it increases in Earth magnetism or decreases in the intensity of the ultraviolet in the sunlight that reaches the ground?

As geomagnetism works better overall than ultraviolet for explaining this grouping of cancer deaths, this would seem to reopen the matter of which might provide the best explanation. To repeat an important idea from the previous chapter, the foundation of this competition was based on the possibility that the northern pattern might possibly be explained "in reality" by one of the explanations rather than by both.

This is particularly the case because both geomagnetism and ultraviolet are correlated very highly together with a value of over .9 (out of 1), the negative direction of that correlation not relevant right now (corr. [geomag08] and [uv0614] = -.902). This high correlation raises the possibility that the statistical results might not be able to distinguish between the two in a way that is meaningful in the real world.

Despite evidence for each of the two leading candidates, the careful analysis in the last chapter about the eight northern cancers persuaded me that the possibility of ultraviolet is the stronger of the two – the weakening sun as we travel north. It is for this reason that I decided to present the ultraviolet model as the final one.

One more piece of evidence, from the model soon to be presented here, added to my final decision. The very fact that I was able to construct a reasonable model for deaths from cancer less lung [canolung] using the numbers for ultraviolet provided additional evidence that ultraviolet could well be the "real" connection to this geographic pattern of dying from cancer.

It is by no means automatic that a model comes out the way one wants. It is quite common that the numbers simply do not "cooperate". While anyone who has tried to do such models knows this to be the case, I thought it was worth mentioning explicitly.

Finally now, we are ready to present the new, simpler model for deaths from cancer less lung. We start with the death rate list in Table 19-1 canolung. Cancer no lung. Death rates from cancer of all kinds in 2010-2012 minus death rates from lung cancer during those same years. [can1012]-[lung1012].

Utah has the fewest deaths of the 51 so called states with about 122 deaths (per hundred thousand people). West Virginia has the most with about 218 deaths. Compared with Utah, the death rate in West Virginia is higher by this much. 121.5/100=217.6/x. 121.5x=21760. X=21760/121.5=179. It is 79 percent higher.

On the low end (fewer deaths) are states including Texas, California, Nevada, Washington DC ("District") and Hawaii. New York is in the lower half with fewer deaths (per hundred thousand people). Rhode Island is in the upper half (more deaths) as are Vermont, Florida, Pennsylvania and Maine. Of course, as we shall soon see, the percent seniors probably affects these numbers greatly so there is not too much we can learn from them.

Next, we can become familiar with the three items that help to explain this pattern after a quick introduction. Age 65, older age, is an important item in the model. More seniors, more deaths from all cancers less lung.

Ultraviolet is the next item. The weaker the ultraviolet in sunlight reaching the ground in the largest city of the state, the more deaths from cancer less lung.

The third and final item is dentist, the percent of the population who said they visited the dentist over the past year. The more who visited the dentist in a state, the fewer who died of cancer of all types with the exception of lung.

The state list for older age can be found in Table 19-2 [age65in6]. Age 65 in 2006. Percent seniors in a state in 2006. Alaska has the lowest percent seniors at about 7 percent while Florida has the highest, at about 17 percent.

Ultraviolet can be found in Table 19-3 [uvi0614]. Average yearly UV Index 2006-2014 for largest city in the state. (Data from NOAA). [They decide to use Baltimore MD for Washington DC (District) to fill in a missing value]. This is the average yearly intensity of ultraviolet in sunlight reaching the ground when the sun is highest in the sky in the largest city of the state. It is over a nine year period including 2006 to 2014. (Typically, the sun gets "weaker" as you go north). It goes from a low UVI (UV Index) value in Alaska of about 2 over the year, to a high in Hawaii of about 11.

Table 19-1 canolung. Cancer no lung. Death rates from cancer of all kinds in 2010- 2012 minus death rates from lung cancer during those same years. [can1012]-[lung1012].

Utah	121.5	New Jersey	184.5
Alaska	122.8	Montana	186.0
Colorado	141.6	South Carolina	187.0
Texas	147.6	Indiana	187.6
Georgia	152.0	Tennessee	188.2
California	154.5	Louisiana	188.2
Nevada	158.5	Oregon	188.4
District	161.7	Rhode Island	189.6
Hawaii	162.2	Delaware	189.7
Virginia	163.6	Missouri	190.1
Arizona	165.9	Wisconsin	190.4
Washington	167.1	Kentucky	191.1
Idaho	167.5	Alabama	192.2
New Mexico	168.7	Michigan	192.4
Maryland	169.4	Oklahoma	193.1
Wyoming	169.7	South Dakota	193.8
North Carolina	172.6	Vermont	195.6
New York	173.7	Arkansas	196.3
Minnesota	175.8	Mississippi	197.6
North Dakota	178.7	Florida	197.6
Illinois	179.1	Ohio	199.8
Massachusetts	181.4	Iowa	199.9
Kansas	181.5	Pennsylvania	212.1
New Hampshire	182.0	Maine	214.8
Connecticut	182.3	West Virginia	217.6
Nebraska	183.0		

Table 19-2 [age65in6].
Age 65 in 2006. Percent seniors in a state in 2006

State	%	State	%
Alaska	6.8	Kansas	12.9
Utah	8.8	New Jersey	12.9
Georgia	9.8	Oregon	12.9
Texas	9.9	Wisconsin	13.0
Colorado	10.0	New York	13.1
California	10.8	Oklahoma	13.2
Nevada	11.1	Missouri	13.3
Idaho	11.5	Nebraska	13.3
Washington	11.5	Massachusetts	13.3
Virginia	11.6	Vermont	13.3
Maryland	11.6	Alabama	13.4
Illinois	12.0	Delaware	13.4
Minnesota	12.1	Connecticut	13.4
Louisiana	12.2	Ohio	13.4
Wyoming	12.2	Montana	13.8
North Carolina	12.2	Arkansas	13.9
District	12.3	Rhode Island	13.9
New Mexico	12.4	Hawaii	14.0
Mississippi	12.4	South Dakota	14.2
Indiana	12.4	Iowa	14.6
New Hampshire	12.4	North Dakota	14.6
Michigan	12.5	Maine	14.6
Tennessee	12.7	Pennsylvania	15.2
Arizona	12.8	West Virginia	15.3
South Carolina	12.8	Florida	16.8
Kentucky	12.8		

Table 19-3 [uvi0614]. Average yearly UV Index 2006-2014 for largest city in the state. (Data from NOAA). [They decide to use Baltimore MD for Washington DC (District) to fill in missing value].

State	UV	State	UV
Alaska	1.9	West Virginia	4.6
Washington	3.5	Missouri	4.8
Oregon	3.6	Kentucky	4.8
Vermont	3.6	Idaho	4.9
Minnesota	3.9	Kansas	5.2
North Dakota	3.9	Virginia	5.4
Maine	3.9	North Carolina	5.4
New Hampshire	4.0	Wyoming	5.5
Michigan	4.0	Tennessee	5.5
Wisconsin	4.1	Oklahoma	5.6
Illinois	4.2	Arkansas	5.6
Massachusetts	4.2	Utah	5.7
Connecticut	4.2	Colorado	5.8
Rhode Island	4.2	Georgia	6.0
South Dakota	4.2	Nevada	6.3
Ohio	4.2	South Carolina	6.3
Iowa	4.3	Mississippi	6.4
New York	4.4	Texas	6.9
Montana	4.4	Arizona	6.9
Pennsylvania	4.4	California	7.0
Nebraska	4.5	New Mexico	7.0
Indiana	4.5	Alabama	7.0
District	4.6	Louisiana	7.2
Maryland	4.6	Florida	8.5
New Jersey	4.6	Hawaii	11.1
Delaware	4.6		

Table 19-4 [dentlvis]. Dental Visits.
Percent of the population in a state visiting the dentist over the past year.

State	%	State	%
West Virginia	53.1	Arizona	68.9
Mississippi	57.1	California	69.0
Oklahoma	57.8	Colorado	69.2
Arkansas	58.5	Oregon	70.2
Louisiana	58.9	Pennsylvania	70.2
Nevada	59.2	Illinois	70.6
Alabama	60.1	Iowa	70.8
Kentucky	60.2	Alaska	71.1
Missouri	60.8	Delaware	71.1
Texas	61.7	New York	71.2
North Dakota	62.9	District	71.4
New Mexico	64.2	Vermont	71.7
Montana	64.3	Maryland	71.9
Georgia	64.7	Nebraska	72.4
Wyoming	65.4	Minnesota	72.9
Idaho	65.7	New Hampshire	72.9
Ohio	66.6	Utah	72.9
Indiana	66.6	Virginia	73.1
South Dakota	66.9	New Jersey	73.6
Kansas	67.0	Rhode Island	75.4
South Carolina	67.0	Wisconsin	75.5
North Carolina	67.1	Massachusetts	75.9
Maine	67.2	Hawaii	77.0
Tennessee	67.5	Michigan	78.0
Washington	67.9	Connecticut	79.1
Florida	68.8		

The third and final item is dentist in Table 19-4 [dentlvis]. Dental Visits. Percent of the population in a state visiting the dentist over the past year. The low is in West Virginia where about 53 percent saw the dentist. The high is in Connecticut where about 79 percent visited.

The final model for death rates from cancer of all kinds except lung [canolung] can be found in Table 19-5. As is the pattern throughout, we begin with the bottom box of correlations to make sure the three items are largely uncorrelated, important to check to avoid erroneous results. The numbers are all low perhaps with the exception of the link between dentist and ultraviolet (-.214). While not perfect, it is still relatively low and uncorrelated (no stars). Having dentist in the model, an extra, improves the model somewhat by revealing a better connection between ultraviolet and cancer deaths.

While down here, we check the bottom line showing a strong link between older age and cancer deaths. For the other two items, we must first wait for the effect of age to be set aside before we can view their true impact, which happens in the final model.

In the top box of Table 19-5, we find the Adjusted R Square of .818, with the model explaining 81.8 percent of the pattern of difference in cancer death rates between states. That is good although, as is typical, much of this is due to the large connection between older age and dying from cancer.

Now we move to the middle box where we find the actual model. As usual, we begin with the two boxes on the right to check statistical significance. In general terms, this is an indicator of the solidness of the results.

For both older age and ultraviolet, Sig. is .000, very good. For dentist, Sig. is .001, not perfect but still good. This result is well below the cutoff of .01, the value I have chosen to use in this research to help ensure that the results are solid.

In the next column, the t value, from which the Sig. value is calculated, is very high for age. We need a minimum of 2 but here, it is over 14. For ultraviolet, it is also high with a value of over 4. For Dentist, it is over 3, all good, suggesting the results are solid.

A glance at the Beta column, whose numbers can be directly compared with each other, reveals that older age is the biggest item contributing to the success of the model. To know the exact contribution of each to the portion of the explanation that the model succeeded to uncover, we do the following.

We add the three numbers together (ignoring decimals and signs) to get a denominator. 867+276+211=1354.

Table 19-5 The Model for all deaths from cancer between 2010 and 2012 with the Exception of Lung Cancer: A Possible Role for Insufficiently strong Ultraviolet in Sunlight:

Model Summary

Model	R	R Square	Adjusted R Square	Std. Error of the Estimate
1	.910[a]	.829	.818	8.5608

a. Predictors: (Constant), DENTLVIS, AGE65IN6, UVI0614

Coefficients[a]

Model		Unstandardized Coefficients		Standardized Coefficients	t	Sig.
		B	Std. Error	Beta		
1	(Constant)	115.886	18.519		6.258	.000
	AGE65IN6	10.412	.728	.867	14.307	.000
	UVI0614	-3.728	.836	-.276	-4.462	.000
	DENTLVIS	-.723	.212	-.211	-3.419	.001

a. Dependent Variable: CANOLUNG

Correlations

		AGE65IN6	UVI0614	DENTLVIS	CANOLUNG
AGE65IN6	Pearson Correlation	1	.090	-.065	.856**
	Sig. (2-tailed)	.	.531	.653	.000
	N	51	51	51	51
UVI0614	Pearson Correlation	.090	1	-.214	-.153
	Sig. (2-tailed)	.531	.	.132	.283
	N	51	51	51	51
DENTLVIS	Pearson Correlation	-.065	-.214	1	-.208
	Sig. (2-tailed)	.653	.132	.	.143
	N	51	51	51	51
CANOLUNG	Pearson Correlation	.856**	-.153	-.208	1
	Sig. (2-tailed)	.000	.283	.143	.
	N	51	51	51	51

**. Correlation is significant at the 0.01 level (2-tailed).

The portion of the model's success that can be attributed to older age is 867/1354=.64 or 64 percent. The portion that can be attributed to ultraviolet is 276/1354=.204 or 20.4 percent. The portion that can be attributed to dentist is 211/1354=.156 or 15.6 percent.

It is perhaps more interesting to know the contribution of each item to the total possible explanation. We know from the Adjusted R Square that the old denominator represents only 81.8 percent of the explanation so we now calculate a new denominator for 100 percent of the explanation, the part the model uncovered as well as the smaller part that was not uncovered. 1354/.818=x/1.   .818x=1354.   X=1354/.818=1655.26.   This is the new denominator.

Of the total possible explanation, older age accounts for 867/1655.26=.524 or 52.4 percent. Ultraviolet accounts for 276/1655.26=.167 or 16.7 percent of the total explanation. Dentist accounts for 211/1655.26=.127 or 12.7 percent of this total explanation.

We are now ready to look at the actual equation in the B column which is a numerical summary of the entire model. This summary is the best attempt to explain, in summary number form, the death rate pattern in the original cancer list in Table 19-1. Here, we will now use this equation to manipulate the result in such a way as to create a "best view" predicted list of deaths from cancer of all kinds minus lung.

We will do this by holding constant the items we find less interesting as a way of getting a better view of the effect of the items we do find interesting. For the items we hold constant, we replace the actual values for each state by the average of all the states. For the items of interest that we allow to vary, we use the actual state values.

We do this by writing the equation from the B column with the above instructions. The statistical software program follows our instructions by plugging in the average value for the items we specify and the actual value for each state when we specify that.

Now comes the hard part, making the decisions which would lead us to the most meaningful view of death rates from cancer minus lung. Surely, we should hold constant older age. We are waiting to see what the pattern looks like after setting aside this large effect but one that is less interesting to us. Second, we surely want to let ultraviolet vary as we are very interested to see its effect.

The big question right now is what to do about dentist. On the one hand, visiting the dentist is something interesting, linked as it is with smoking. The more smokers, the fewer who visited the dentist. The correlation between dentist [dentlvis] and smoking [smokdali] is minus -.437**.

I suspect that visiting the dentist, and the posited better oral hygiene at home which results, might be an important part of the cancer story. It might implicate the buildup of dangerous mouth bacteria as involved with cancer when oral hygiene is neglected.

On the other hand, however, our focus right now is on this "north" pattern, the observation that more people die from cancer as we drive north. Given that focus, it seems clear to me (now) that we should hold constant the dentist item, however intrinsically interesting it is. This is in order to focus right now on "north". We will do that by using the average value for the percent of the population who visited the dentist. This leaves us with only ultraviolet to vary.

Thus, we need two numbers for averages called means. The mean for older age is 12.653 (percent). The mean for dentist is 67.906 (percent who say they DID visit). With these numbers now in hand, we can write the equation below from the B column in Table 19-5, middle box. We instruct SPSS 11 to run it by selecting transform, compute (from the data file). We will give a name to the resulting list called canouvil. This stands for cancer no lung UVI (UV Index) list. Canouvil = 115.886 + (10.412 * 12.653) − (3.728 * uvi0614) − (.723 * 67.906). I will run this now.

The statistical program "solves" this equation for each state and yields the death list in Table 19-6. Table 19-6 canouvil. Cancer no lung UVI (UV Index) list. Best view predicted death rates from cancer of all types except lung in 2010-2012 based on actual death rates but setting aside the impact of older age (more deaths) and visiting the dentist (fewer deaths) in order to see the effect of weakening ultraviolet in sunlight on increasing death rates. Of course, the order of this list is the same as the list for ultraviolet in Table 19-3 but the direction is reversed. This is because, as ultraviolet goes DOWN, cancer deaths (less lung) go UP.

While Hawaii has the lowest death rate, Florida is second lowest, a pattern that becomes clear only after setting aside older age. California is in that top group of states with the fewest cancer deaths. Arizona and Nevada also do well. New York is in the bottom half (with more predicted deaths) together with New Jersey. Rhode Island is worse (even more deaths).

Table 19-6 canouvil cancer no lung UVI (UV Index) list.
Best view predicted death rate from cancer of all types except lung in 2010-2012 based on actual death rates. Here, we set aside the impact of older age (more deaths) and visiting the dentist (fewer deaths) in order to see the possible effect of weakening ultraviolet in sunlight on increasing death rate:

Hawaii	157.2	Maryland	181.4
Florida	166.8	District	181.4
Louisiana	171.7	New Jersey	181.4
Alabama	172.4	Indiana	181.8
New Mexico	172.4	Nebraska	181.8
California	172.4	Montana	182.1
Arizona	172.8	Pennsylvania	182.1
Texas	172.8	New York	182.1
Mississippi	174.7	Iowa	182.5
South Carolina	175.0	South Dakota	182.9
Nevada	175.0	Illinois	182.9
Georgia	176.2	Connecticut	182.9
Colorado	176.9	Massachusetts	182.9
Utah	177.3	Ohio	182.9
Arkansas	177.7	Rhode Island	182.9
Oklahoma	177.7	Wisconsin	183.2
Wyoming	178.0	Michigan	183.6
Tennessee	178.0	New Hampshire	183.6
North Carolina	178.4	Minnesota	184.0
Virginia	178.4	North Dakota	184.0
Kansas	179.1	Maine	184.0
Idaho	180.3	Vermont	185.1
Missouri	180.6	Oregon	185.1
Kentucky	180.6	Washington	185.5
West Virginia	181.4	Alaska	191.4
Delaware	181.4		

The most predicted deaths from cancer minus lung are in Vermont, Washington (state) and Alaska.

To review briefly, this list is based on the equation which is our best numerical attempt to explain the overall pattern in the 2010-2012 death rates from cancer minus lung in Table 19-1. The state listing varies based on one thing that changes. As the yearly ultraviolet in sunlight gets weaker and weaker (when we travel north), the death rate from these cancers gets higher and higher.

Table 19-6 shows that the lowest predicted death rate is in Hawaii with the strongest ultraviolet, of about 157 deaths per hundred thousand. The highest predicted death rate from cancer minus lung is in Alaska with 191 deaths. Compared with the lowest Hawaii rate, the Alaska rate is how much larger? $157/100=191/x$. $157x=19100$. $X=19100/157$. $X=121.66$. The Alaska rate is higher by about 21.7 percent or a little more than a fifth. This is another way to assess the size of the ultraviolet effect on death rates from cancer less lung. This is slightly larger than the 16.7 percent of the total explanation attributed to variations in ultraviolet calculated earlier.

Now, as a finale, we can return briefly to the matter of interpretation. How does this new model for all deaths from cancer minus lung cancer move forward our understanding? First, it further confirms this northern geographic pattern considerably. More north, more deaths from these cancers. In the last chapter about the eight northern cancers, it included some 49 percent of all deaths (.4894) (based on death rates). Now evidence has been presented that this northern pattern includes almost all the cancer deaths, 100 minus the 27.7 percent of lung cancer deaths which equals 72.3 percent of all deaths from cancer (based on these rates).

There is no reason to stop there, however. In Chapter 3, the lung cancer model also provides evidence that this cancer too, after controls, exhibits a northern pattern. More north, more deaths. In sum, as for "north", this current model here provides the missing portion. We can now conclude that, based on these death rates, all cancer deaths reveal a northern geographic pattern (after accounting for other items). When we travel north, there are more deaths.

As for which environmental factor might best explain this northern geographic pattern, the overall evidence is mixed between the two best ideas from the individual models for each kind of cancer. According to the first, it is increased Earth magnetism as we travel north that might best explain the pattern. According to the second, it is the decreased intensity of ultraviolet reaching the ground in sunlight as we move north.

As I mentioned earlier, this broader model for all cancer deaths less lung suggests that magnetism might be the stronger explanation for this north pattern. And yet, I decided to present the model suggesting that ultraviolet might be the key environmental factor. I was persuaded to take this course in light of the analysis in the previous chapter suggesting that ultraviolet is stronger when those eight cancers are seen together.

As in this earlier chapter, I am of the belief that successfully constructing a model with ultraviolet does add to the plausibility that it may be that after all. That is what was achieved here in the model presented in Table 19-5.

In sum, I believe that the overall thrust of the evidence favors ultraviolet as the best explanation for this northern geographic pattern of cancer deaths uncovered here. This is confirmed for the eight cancers in the last chapter including lung cancer, about which a separate model was constructed in Chapter 3.

While this much broader model here provides contrary evidence (in a model not shown), the success of an ultraviolet-based model lends plausibility to the thesis that it MIGHT be diminished ultraviolet in sunlight that serves as the best explanation for why more people die from cancer as we travel north.

On a final note, I wish to mark the occasion of the completion of the last model in Table 19-5. This model for all cancer deaths less lung cancer includes the three items already noted. We have the necessary control for older age, and then two additional items. These are weaker ultraviolet (more deaths) and not going to the dentist, (more deaths).

The other piece of the cancer story is lung cancer in Chapter 3, Table 3-4. This lung cancer model includes not going to college (more deaths) as a control. It also shows a possible connection with weaker ultraviolet (more deaths from lung cancer). Here, however, the Sig. value is a little less solid at .007.

As a rough summary, these two models together, (all cancer minus lung and then, plus lung cancer) represents all deaths from cancer. Leaving aside the control items (of older age and not attending college), dying from cancer appears linked first with ultraviolet in sunlight that is not strong enough.

It might also be linked with not going to the dentist regularly. In my interpretation, this is probably related to not being diligent enough at home with keeping the teeth clean. This result indirectly suggests the possibility that the buildup of dangerous mouth bacteria might be part of the cancer story.

Understanding the key ultraviolet finding here is not an easy task. In an earlier chapter, I made the argument that any difference in actual exposure from place to place is a poor explanation for the pattern. Of course, I do believe that exposure to sunlight is necessary in order to posit a possible anti-cancer effect. Nevertheless, I feel that the pattern here, of more north - more deaths, must be due to differences in the sun itself that reaches the ground in different places.

There is a greater tilt of the planet away from the sun the more north we travel in the northern hemisphere, where the United States happens to be situated. As a result, the angle of sunlight increases and the sunlight reaching the ground is weaker in intensity. This is surely the case for the ultraviolet portion of sunlight reaching the ground based on the yearly UV Index (UVI).

The statistical evidence here from state death rates of cancer in the United States leads to the following possibility. As the ultraviolet in sunlight weakens, more people die from cancer. This suggests that there might be some role for strong enough ultraviolet in both preventing cancer and fighting it after it has taken hold.

Sources and Acknowledgements

I apologize that the standard detail on sources for data is absent in many cases. This is due, in part, to the years over which this project unfolded. Given the multitude of items I examined after putting them into number form, it might reflect a deficit in my organizing skills for an endeavor of this size.

Most of the cancer death rates are from the Center for Disease Control website, cdc.gov, the Health Data Interactive table. This project closed in July 2016, making it now quite difficult to independently verify the death rate numbers. Given this unexpected development, it is perhaps lucky that I decided to include in the tables the actual death rate for each state as well as numbers by state for each connected "item". While this does not make outside verification any easier, it does make it possible for readers to rerun each model from scratch should they so desire.

All cancer death rates are for adults age 18 and over. There are a few cancer models that use age-adjusted rates done by others. I presume these include deaths among only adults as well.

When it was open, I went to cdc.gov/nchs. Click health data interactive. Click mortality and life expectancy. Click mortality by underlying cause. Age 18+: US/State, 2001-2009 (these death numbers kept being updated). (source: NVSS). I would click right arrow for the first of the 51 "states", recording each state death rate. I typically used numbers (from memory) for 18+ crude, gender all, race all. In later years they started grouping death rates in three year increments, constructing a yearly death rate based on that time period. One random detail from my notes is for melanoma, "malignant melanoma of the skin" IC D-10 code C43.

Two or more of the cancers modeled here were not a part of the Health Data Interactive table and I was forced to settle for whatever numbers I could find from other sources. Typically these are age-adjusted numbers, meaning that the differences in the age of the population from one state to the other were already taken into consideration when producing these rates.

The "items" I used to test for a linkage with the pattern of death rates from each kind of cancer were part of a data base I constructed over the course of many years. They are all on the level of US states (including Washington DC) and are from readily available sources such as the Statistical Abstract of the United States. Examples include demographic items such as older age (65+), college (I chose having attended at least some college), percent black, Jewish, Asian.

Also geographic details needed to calculate geomagnetism on the ground were from online sources. I used a USGS (US Geological Survey) online calculator based on latitude, longitude and different measures for altitude (elevation) for my 51 cities. Other weather related numbers were from both the hard copy and later, the online edition, of a reference book called Weather.

On rare occasions, I acquired special surveys such as one for pet ownership in the United States. It was from this survey that I found numbers on the percent of households with a dog by state.

As I mention numerous times in the text, ultraviolet is captured in number form for the largest city of the state by using a version of the UV Index (UVI), from NOAA, about which there is a wealth of information on their various pages online. As best as I understand, these numbers were aggregated at my request into a yearly rate for each of the cities, on two occasions.

The first was many years ago, in the late 1990s, when Craig Long did this for me for the year 1996 sending the information by fax. In about 2015, I made contact again, and he updated this set of numbers based on a nine year period of 2006-2014, this time sending the new information by an email attachment.

Perhaps noteworthy, this first set of 1996 numbers hinted at some connection between ultraviolet and cancer in the very early years of this project. I realized, however, that I did these models "incorrectly" using in the same model two items (one being ultraviolet) that were highly correlated with each other. Upon learning that this was not allowed, the idea of ultraviolet receded over the course of many years. More recently, I tried it again and during this latter period, the results were both valid and successful.

The ultraviolet numbers proved to be an important key to this project. Perhaps I never could have provided evidence for the connection between insufficiently strong ultraviolet and cancer had I not had the good fortune of acquiring these numbers. While nobody knew how the result would turn out beforehand, I feel a debt of gratitude to the people who created the UV Index in light of the good science behind it.

As I have done several times in the text, I extend my thanks to Craig Long at NOAA for his critical help in aggregating the UV Index (UVI) values from daily into yearly form. As I have also stated frequently, in light of the controversial finding here, I must be clear that those who helped me bear no responsibility for the contrarian nature of the result.

I must also thank Steve Mackin, formerly of solarmeter.com, where I bought my several instruments for measuring sunlight, mainly ultraviolet. Steve was always cheerful and helpful whenever a technical question came up about measuring ultraviolet. I learned a great deal from using these meters which contributed to my overall knowledge on the general subject. Steve now sells personal size meters for measuring sunlight at his site uvmeter.net.

At the end of the breast cancer chapter, I note a measurable decline in air pollution with each passing year. These comments are based on an analysis of air pollution over time in the United States epa.gov/airtrends/aq trends.html. Percent change in air quality 2000 vs. 2013. (Syntax might not be exactly right).

While my measures for (galactic) cosmic radiation never made it directly into the models, at least the topic was discussed in the chapter with the three summary tables. It was in the context of trying to understand how rain is connected with more deaths from cancer.

My understanding of our physical world has much benefited from the time I spent learning about this topic. Some of my numbers on the subject of cosmic radiation in different cities come from a paper written by James Ziegler (and others). Over an extended period, we exchanged occasional emails which were very helpful.

On the related subject of geomagnetic cutoff rigidity, I was in email contact with Margaret (Peggy) A. Shea and Don F. Smart and I feel a sense of gratitude to them for answering my questions and helping to improve my understanding of this feature of cosmic radiation. In the text, I raise the possibility that elevated radiation might be behind the connection between rain and cancer.

In the late 1990s, I made telephone contact with Michael Holick, Ph.D., M.D. to ask him a question and followed up with some emails over the years, mainly on the subject of Vitamin D, that I recall. I thank him for his help.

As a brief technical note, I developed my data set of "items" for testing over a nineteen year period using the statistical software package SPSS. Over most of these years, I used SPSS version 11 (11.0.4) on an Apple laptop running Mac OS X version 10.4.11, Processor 1.33 GHz PowerPC G4.

Most of the tables are exports from my data file to "syntax" files. The tables with actual models are an abridged version of SPSS output removing the boxes, such as Anova, that I do not use. Of course, on this output, I added my own text to serve as a title.

I wish to thank the three Brown professors on my dissertation committee in graduate school years ago for helping to develop my analytic skills: Calvin Goldscheider, Darrell West and my chair, Alan Zuckerman, of blessed memory. I also thank Debra Nelson and Dr. Thomas Allen for both their help with library research and their friendship. Also, I must mention my beloved father, Bob Greenbaum, may he rest in peace. He contributed in many ways to the arrival of this day. Finally, I thank my friend David Reiner, of blessed memory, who volunteered to read the entire manuscript. I miss his kindness and his brilliance.

Copyright Keith Reed Greenbaum, Ph.D.
November 1, 2017
Providence Rhode Island, United States of America

www.ingramcontent.com/pod-product-compliance
Lightning Source LLC
Chambersburg PA
CBHW052342220526
45465CB00003BA/915